How Nursing has Changed with Technology

Editor

MARIA OVERSTREET

NURSING CLINICS OF NORTH AMERICA

www.nursing.theclinics.com

Consulting Editor
STEPHEN D. KRAU

June 2015 • Volume 50 • Number 2

ELSEVIER

1600 John F. Kennedy Boulevard • Suite 1800 • Philadelphia, Pennsylvania, 19103-2899

http://www.theclinics.com

NURSING CLINICS OF NORTH AMERICA Volume 50, Number 2
June 2015 ISSN 0029-6465, ISBN-13: 978-0-323-38896-2

Editor: Kerry Holland
Developmental Editor: Casey Jackson

Nursing Clinics of North America (ISSN 0029-6465) is published quarterly by Elsevier Inc., 360 Park Avenue South, New York, NY 10010-1710. Months of issue are March, June, September, and December. Periodicals postage paid at New York, NY and additional mailing offices. Subscription price per year is, $150.00 (US individuals), $400.00 (US institutions), $275.00 (international individuals), $488.00 (international institutions), $220.00 (Canadian individuals), $488.00 (Canadian institutions), $85.00 (US students), and $135.00 (international students). To receive student/resident rate, orders must be accompanied by name of affiliated institution, date of term, and the signature of program/residency coordinator on institution letterhead. Orders will be billed at individual rate until proof of status is received. Foreign air speed delivery is included in all *Clinics* subscription prices. All prices are subject to change without notice. **POSTMASTER:** Send address changes to *Nursing Clinics*, Elsevier Health Sciences Division, Subscription Customer Service, 3251 Riverport Lane, Maryland Heights, MO 63043. **Customer Service: Telephone: 1-800-654-2452** (U.S. and Canada); **1-314-447-8871 (outside U.S. and Canada). Fax: 1-314-447-8029. E-mail: journalscustomerservice-usa@elsevier.com** (for print support) and **journalsonlinesupport-usa@elsevier.com** (for online support).

Nursing Clinics of North America is covered in *EMBASE/Excerpta Medica, MEDLINE/PubMed (Index Medicus), Social Sciences Citation Index, Current Contents, ASCA, Cumulative Index to Nursing, RNdex Top 100,* and Allied Health Literature and International Nursing Index (INI).

Contributors

CONSULTING EDITOR

STEPHEN D. KRAU, PhD, RN, CNE
Associate Professor, Vanderbilt University Medical Center, School of Nursing, Nashville, Tennessee

EDITOR

MARIA OVERSTREET, PhD, RN
Professor, Director of Center for Clinical Simulation, Director of Student Services, Middle Tennessee School of Anesthesia, Madison, Tennessee; Associate Professor of Nursing, Vanderbilt University School of Nursing, Nashville, Tennessee

AUTHORS

CASSANDRA BERGERO, MSN, CNS, FNP
Director of Patient Safety and Infection Control, Center for Quality and Clinical Effectiveness, Lucile Packard Children's Hospital at Stanford, Palo Alto, California

RACHEL M. BROWN, CRNA, DNP
Assistant Program Administrator, Middle Tennessee School of Anesthesia, Madison, Tennessee

DAVID M. DIPERSIO, PharmD
Vanderbilt University Medical Center, Nashville, Tennessee

KRISA HOYLE ELGIN, MSN, FNP, MPH
Director of Research and Innovation, Center for Quality and Clinical Effectiveness; Cardiac Anesthesia Nurse Practitioner, Lucile Packard Children's Hospital at Stanford, Palo Alto, California

FRANCISCA CISNEROS FARRAR, EdD, MSN, RN
Professor, School of Nursing, Austin Peay State University, Clarksville, Tennessee

AMY C. GIDEON, MS, EdD
Director of Institutional Effectiveness and Learning Resources, Middle Tennessee School of Anesthesia, Madison, Tennessee

BETH F. HALLMARK, PhD, RN
College of Health Sciences, Belmont University, Nashville, Tennessee

MELANIE R. KEIFFER, DNP, ANP-BC, CCRN
Assistant Professor, College of Nursing and Health, Madonna University, Livonia, Michigan; Nurse Practitioner, Advanced Practice Provider Services, Henry Ford West Bloomfield Hospital, West Bloomfield Township, Michigan

CHRISTIAN KETEL DNP, RN
Instructor of Clinical Nursing, Clinical Practice and Community Partnerships, Vanderbilt University School of Nursing, Nashville, Tennessee

STEPHEN D. KRAU, PhD, RN, CNE
Associate Professor, Vanderbilt University Medical Center, School of Nursing, Nashville, Tennessee

SUSAN KRAUSER LUPEAR, DNP, CRNA, APRN
Interim Chief CRNA, Vanderbilt University Medical Center, Nashville, Tennessee

LEWIS McCARVER, DNP, CRNA
Professor and Instructor in Clinical Simulation, Middle Tennessee School of Anesthesia, Madison, Tennessee

SALLY MILLER, MS, RN
Assistant Professor of Nursing and Manager, Clinical Learning Center, Vanderbilt University School of Nursing, Nashville, Tennessee

MINDY MCCALLUM MULLINS, CRNA, DNAP
Department of Anesthesia, Baptist Memorial Hospital North Mississippi, Oxford, Mississippi

MARIA OVERSTREET, PhD, RN
Professor, Director of Center for Clinical Simulation, Director of Student Services, Middle Tennessee School of Anesthesia, Madison, Tennessee; Associate Professor of Nursing, Vanderbilt University School of Nursing, Nashville, Tennessee

JORDAN PATTERSON, BA
Instructional Technology Specialist, Middle Tennessee School of Anesthesia, Madison, Tennessee

JOHN SHIELDS, DNP, CRNA
Professor and Instructor in Clinical Simulation, Cardiac Anesthesia Division, Department of Anesthesiology, Vanderbilt University Medical Center, Nashville, Tennessee; Professor, Middle Tennessee School of Anesthesia, Madison, Tennessee

BENJAMIN A. SMALLHEER, PhD, RN, ACNP-BC, CCRN
Assistant Professor of Nursing, Vanderbilt University School of Nursing; Acute Care Nurse Practitioner, Pulmonary Intensivist/Rapid Response Team, St. Thomas West Hospital, Nashville, Tennessee

Contents

> Bedside technology pressures nurses to integrate and master a variety of new tools, devices, and methods of monitoring patient status. We review opportunities and challenges in the relationship between bedside nursing and technology. The increasing amount of available technology has impacted bedside nurses. The relationship between bedside nursing and technology is largely positive. Big data holds great potential for translating digital patient information into expanded knowledge tools for the bedside nurse, the development of which require nursing involvement. More research is needed to explore the concept of the nurse as advocate in high-technology patient care.

> With the prevalence of obesity escalating globally, an increasing number of patients who are obese are seeking elective or requiring emergency surgery. Certified registered nurse anesthetists are challenged to provide vigilant, safe care. The ability to provide supportive therapy and make anesthetic adjustments is often hindered with obesity. Although technological advancements may enhance patient care delivery, health care providers must question why and how specific tasks are performed. Health care providers should challenge themselves to acquire and evaluate current evidence that enables communication with colleagues, dissemination of findings to health care providers worldwide, and implementation of evidence-based practice.

> Hospital technology has aggressively improved over the past 50 years. With the primary intent of making health care more efficient and safer, the bedside nurse has been impacted by all of these changes. The growth and utilization of point-of-care testing, automated dispensing systems, electronic medication records, electronic health records, mobile and digital radiography, and computerized provider order entry have continued to foster the growth of Nursing autonomy and the expectation of nurses'

critical thinking. The usability and utility of these advancing technologies are key components to end-user satisfaction and ultimately the adoption of the technology by the bedside nurse.

Telehealth technology is an evidence-based delivery model tool that can be integrated into the plan of care for mental health patients. Telehealth technology empowers access to health care, can help decrease or prevent hospital readmissions, assist home health nurses provide shared decision making, and focuses on collaborative care. Telehealth and the recovery model have transformed the role of the home health nurse. Nurses need to be proactive and respond to rapidly emerging technologies that are transforming their role in home care.

Internet-based applications and mobile health technology has advanced at unprecedented rates over the last decade and has proved to be a highly effective platform for communication. Simultaneously, the United States health care system has reached a critical and unsustainable level of spending, arising largely from ingrained system inefficiencies and overall suboptimum communication. Internet-based and mobile health technology offers an innovative solution to both of these problems. The prevention of readmissions for heart failure provides an excellent example of how this new technology can be used in today's health care environment to improve patient care.

Preventable adverse events and other medical errors occur to hundreds of thousands of Americans every year. The financial burden of these preventable events is estimated to be $29 billion. According to the World Health Organization, reducing medical errors has become an international concern. Protecting patients from harm is a primary responsibility of all nurses regardless of whether the nurse works in the intensive care unit or operating room. Adherence to policies to maintain patient safety can be discerned once the level of knowledge of these policies among nurses is determined.

The Health Information Technology for Economic and Clinical Health (HI-TECH) Act has greatly increased the acceptance of electronic health record technology by providing incentives and punishment standards. A key criterion of the HITECH Act, meaningful use, has vendors clamoring to design clinical decision support (CDS) systems that fulfill this objective.

Users should be aware that more emphasis may be placed on achieving the goals for compliance than on working out details that are clinically meaningful. Nurses can play a crucial rule in collaboratively supporting CDS initiative changes that make patient care more effective and efficient.

Melanie R. Keiffer

Clinical practice guidelines augment clinician decision making. Researchers cite a lack of knowledge of guideline existence, complexity of guidelines, staff attitude, lack of training, time and resource constraints as reasons for nonadherence. This project sought to understand factors that promote or prevent guideline implementation at the point of care. Respondents' viewed clinical practice guidelines as valid tools necessary to standardize patient care and exhibited proficiency in synthesis and integration of guidelines into clinical decisions and treatment plans. Efficient and effective guidelines impact patient safety and quality by increasing the consistency of behavior and replacing idiosyncratic behaviors with best practices.

Maria Overstreet, Lewis McCarver, John Shields, and Jordan Patterson

Videos of hand-off and initial assessment (Video 1); recruitment of the surgeon, hemodynamic manipulation, and fluid administration; communication and hypotension (Video 2) after declamping; provider collaboration and handover (Video 3); conclusion of the scenario and debriefing (Video 4) accompany this article

The use of simulation technology has introduced a challenge for simulation nurse educators: evaluation of student performance. The subjectivity of student performance evaluation has been in need of improvement. It is imperative to provide clear and consistent information to the learner of expectations for their performance. Educators use objectives to define for the learner what the primary focus will be in the learning activities. Creation of rubrics to replace checklists to evaluate learner performance is a team task. Improved rubrics assist instructors in providing valuable, immediate, and postactivity feedback and consistency among instructors, and improved inter-rater reliability.

Sally Miller and Maria Overstreet

According to the Centers for Disease Control and Prevention, patients age 65 and older account for 43% of hospital days. The complexity of caring for older adults affords nursing students opportunities to assess, prioritize, intervene, advocate, and experience being a member of an interdisciplinary health care team. However, these multifaceted hospital experiences are not consistently available for all students. Nursing clinical simulation (NCS) can augment or replace specific clinical hours and provide clinically relevant experiences to practice management and leadership skills while caring for older adults. This article describes a geriatric management and leadership NCS.

The complexity of the relationship between nursing and technology is not new. The complexity has increased with the advent of new technology and technological devices. For faculty who are in the clinical area on a limited basis, and for nurses who are not involved in decisions related to the adoption of technology, terms and concepts related to technology can be misconstrued or misunderstood. An overview of some major terms used in reference to technology and technological approaches can only enhance the intricate relationship between nursing and technology.

Over the past 10 years, education in nursing has changed and simulation is a new teaching technology being used. Unfortunately, lack of training of how to use simulation in education can translate into poor educational pedagogy. This article introduces the importance of training educators and clinicians to use simulation technology according to defined standards and recommendations. A literature search revealed a dearth of research related to faculty training. Described are some programs in place across the United States that have been developed to facilitate education of faculty in use of simulation technology and methodology.

Advances in technology have assisted in the proliferation of short-term, faith-based international medical mission trips. Many of these mission trips include health care not only to local citizens but also building schools and churches and sharing the Gospel of Jesus Christ. Included in this article are my own personal experiences in short-term, faith-based medical missions. A step-by-step guide is offered to help prepare inexperienced mission participants gain insight into short-term mission trips. Advanced planning, fundraising, collaboration, and being open to change are key elements to successful participation in these life-changing missions.

Despite focused attention to improve the quality and safety of patient care, and the financial impact pressure ulcers (PUs) can have on a health care provider or institution, evidence supports that PUs continue to occur in other patient populations during admission to the hospital. An example of a patient population in which evidence indicates that the development of PUs occurs, is patients who have a surgical procedure. The article discusses a project designed to identify potential knowledge deficits among perioperative nurses of indicators for PU development in the surgical patient population.

NURSING CLINICS OF NORTH AMERICA

THE CLINICS ARE AVAILABLE ONLINE!
Access your subscription at:
www.theclinics.com

Foreword

Technology in Nursing: The Mandate for New Implementation and Adoption Approaches

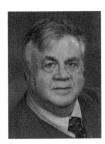

Stephen D. Krau, PhD, RN, CNE
Consulting Editor

The advances of technology in health care and nursing remain one of the fastest growing aspects of our profession. As technology explodes on the health care scene, the technological rift between nursing skills, knowledge, and terminology increases. Use of technology in so many aspects of our profession is unavoidable and is well supported by the Institute of Medicine. In their report in 2011, *The Future of Nursing: Leading Change, Advancing Health*, there is an explicit recommendation that health care organizations, in addition to "private and public funders [to] collaborate to advance research on innovative solutions, including technology that will enable nurses to contribute to improved health care."[1] The report recommends that health care organizations employ "frontline staff in design, development, purchase, implementation, and evaluation of 'devices and technology products'."[1,2]

The focus of technological advances in health care is to directly improve the delivery of patient care in health care facilities. Technology is used to diagnose patients, monitor patients, treat patients, record information about patients, as well as to facilitate earlier discharges for patients.[2] Implications for utilization go far beyond the beside, as they impact budget and have important ramifications for traditional nursing education as well as staff development. The continual infusion of technology into all venues of health care requires thoughtful consideration, as there is limited understanding of how health care facilities make decisions about, procure, embrace, and ultimately, implement technology.

As identified by Schoville and Titler from the University of Michigan, there are two main spheres of models and theories that are related to the use of technology. These include technology adoption and the sciences of implementation.[2] Technology

http://dx.doi.org/10.1016/j.cnur.2015.03.011
0029-6465/15/$ – see front matter © 2015 Published by Elsevier Inc.
nursing.theclinics.com

adoption primarily refers to how the technology is adopted by the parties that will be using it. Technology implementation is concerned with methods, interventions, and variables that encourage the use of evidence-based practice.[2] These two areas remain somewhat isolated from one another and do not articulate well in practice. With energies being focused on the use of the technology, it is not hard to understand how other considerations related to technology and its use remain unstudied. There is a multitude of factors at multiple levels that impact the success of technology implementation.[3] These factors become more involved as the technology and choices related to technology become more complex.

As we venture forward in the twenty-first century, it has become as much of an imperative to study methods in which technology is adopted as well as how the implementation informs the use of technology. Research into these domains will need to include a broader focus, including vendors, economics, and regulation agencies. Already with the impetus of "meaningful use" reimbursement for clinical health care records, it is easy to see how more incentives will emerge. It is hoped that the newer incentives will consider issues that patients perceive as important, and not necessarily what political leaders consider important. As technology moves forward, models such as those created by Schoville and Titler will form the basis for further consideration and it is hoped, bridge the gap in current technology adoption and sciences of implementation. As rapidly as technology advances, models and theories related to technology implementation and adoption cannot remain stagnant.

Stephen D. Krau, PhD, RN, CNE
Vanderbilt University Medical Center
School of Nursing
461 21st Avenue, South
Nashville, TN 37240, USA

E-mail address:
steve.krau@vanderbilt.edu

REFERENCES

1. Institute of Medicine. The future of nursing: leading change, advancing health. Washington, DC: National Academies Press; 2011.
2. Schoville RR, Titler MG. Guiding healthcare technology implementation: a new integrated technology implementation model. Comput Inform Nurs 2015;33(3): 99–107.
3. Durlak J, DuPre EP. Implementation matters: a review of research on the influence of implementation of program outcomes and the factors affecting implementation. Am J Community Psychol 2008;41:327–50.

Preface

Transforming Nursing Practice with Technology

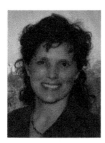

Maria Overstreet, PhD, RN
Editor

Several facets of nursing practice are constants. Two such facets that have not changed over time are nurses as patient advocates as well as nurses practicing the art of caring. In some areas of nursing practice, especially in the delivery of state-of-the-art bedside nursing care, changes have evolved. The availability of technology at the bedside has been instrumental in these changes. For example, nurse educators have begun to change educational methods to engage students, nurses in current practice, as well as patients, families, and even communities.

In this issue, you will hear from nursing experts about their research, quality improvement projects, and personal experiences regarding changes in the delivery of nursing care. Nursing experts will describe how the use of technology has changed their practice, how technology has improved patient discharge into the outpatient setting, how monitoring of patients has improved with technology, and how technology has made it easier to educate, use survey tools, and implement quality improvement projects. These experts will also warn us about using technology just because we can. You will read about a project by Mullins, who warns about the simple task of blood pressure monitoring with an obese population and the implications for nurse anesthetists perioperatively. You will also be intrigued by the creativity of some of the reports of nursing quality improvement projects implemented easily due to the changes in technology.

I believe this issue is important for all nurses to read, and I believe the adoption of new technological advancements is now part of the foundation of nursing practice. It is good practice to keep abreast of changes occurring in other disciplines as well as in our own so that we may apply others' successes to our own specific areas of nursing. Informatics in nursing is a growing field and nursing as a whole must embrace technology and learn to adapt various methods of delivery so that we can appropriately care for and advocate for all our patients.

Nurs Clin N Am 50 (2015) xiii–xiv
http://dx.doi.org/10.1016/j.cnur.2015.03.010
0029-6465/15/$ – see front matter © 2015 Published by Elsevier Inc.

nursing.theclinics.com

We are beginning to see the closing of a circle of care. Our roots began in the home; then we transformed to the acute care setting, and now we are in the beginning stages of transforming back to providing care for the patient and family in the home or community setting because of new advances in technology such as telehealth and ihealth. With the changes in our national health care system, we must encourage all nurses to be entrepreneurial and to incorporate new methods of care delivery as well as encourage ideas of how nursing can improve.

I encourage you to engage with the article that resonates with your practice and discuss your thoughts with these expert nurses. You are the success of nursing and you will make a difference!

Maria Overstreet, PhD, RN
Middle Tennessee School of Anesthesia
315 Hospital Drive
Madison, TN 37116, USA

Vanderbilt University School of Nursing
Nashville, TN 37240, USA

E-mail address:
m.overstreet@mtsa.edu

Technology and the Bedside Nurse

An Exploration and Review of Implications for Practice

Krisa Hoyle Elgin, MSN, FNP, MPH*, Cassandra Bergero, MSN, CNS, FNP

KEYWORDS

- Technology • High reliability • Quality of care • Patient safety • Patient care
- Patient experience • Big data

KEY POINTS

- Nursing has a well-established history of successfully deploying and integrating patient care technology.
- The accelerating pace of technological developments and devices in health care challenges nursing to balance the demands of learning new technology with maintaining the patient at the center of care.
- Health care–related technologies such as the electronic medical record have shown clear evidence that they are associated with improved nursing-sensitive patient outcomes.
- Nursing involvement is needed to develop new, nursing-focused patient care technology and optimize technology already in place.
- The role of the bedside nurse as advocate for patients is taking on new and uncharted dimensions in the age of technology.

INTRODUCTION

Nursing has been successfully designing, organizing and guiding the patient's experiences and expectations of health care technology since the late 1700s.[1]

> ...A true creator is necessity, which is the mother of our invention.
> —Plato, an excerpt from The Republic, 369BC.

Disclosure Statement: K.H. Elgin is grant funded by Hewlett Packard Labs.
Center for Quality and Clinical Effectiveness, Lucile Packard Children's Hospital at Stanford, 700 Welch Road, Suite 225, Palo Alto, CA 94304, USA
* Corresponding author.
E-mail address: KElgin@stanfordchildrens.org

Nurs Clin N Am 50 (2015) 227–239
http://dx.doi.org/10.1016/j.cnur.2015.02.001
0029-6465/15/$ – see front matter © 2015 Elsevier Inc. All rights reserved.

nursing.theclinics.com

Some of the initial technological wonders that nurses either developed or widely integrated into clinical practice include the measuring spoon, thermometer, flexible urinary catheter, hospital bed, and syringe. By including these and other devices in patient care, nurses acted as a catalyzing force in the early technological transformation of health care in the United States.

> *Everything that can be invented, has been invented.*
> *—A quote from 1899 by Charles H. Duell, commissioner of the U.S. patent office.*

Around the turn of the 20th century, the role of nursing in shaping medical technology became progressively more visible.[2] As new technologies accumulated in hospitals and patient care areas, nurses were charged with mastering them.[3,4] By the mid 1900s, the pace of technological development in the health sector had increased significantly, as had the development of formal nursing education programs and the number of hospitals in America.[5]

> *I think there is a worldwide market for maybe five computers.*
> *—A now famous quote made by IBM president Thomas J. Watson in 1943.*

In 1991, a new and uncharted era of possibility for technology and human health emerged when the Human Genome Project began and the world wide web was launched. Since then, the fields of biotechnology, genetic medicine, and digital health data have grown with unimaginable speed, spread and application.[6] As the Internet and the electronic medical record (EMR) expanded, patients gradually and increasingly gained access to their own information, as well as to treatment options surrounding impending health care decisions, symptoms, or medications. As a result, the way that patients, clinicians, and the health system as a whole connect to, process, and utilize information is evolving, as are the expectations of what technology can deliver.

> *Any sufficiently designed technology is indistinguishable from magic.*
> *—A quote by Arthur C. Clark, one of the world's best-selling authors of science fiction.*

At 3 million licensed members, registered nurses comprise the largest professional group within the health care system.[7] It follows that nurses, along with their patients, are the 2 groups impacted at the point of care by technology. The nursing literature demonstrates wide variation in how nurses perceive and receive the impact that technology has on their practice.[8–10] Similarly variable is the description of nursing's adjustment to the ever-increasing amount of technology in the patient care setting.[11,12] Although there is less literature describing how nursing is influencing the technology that is driving massive change in the patient care environment, there is no doubt that technology has been, and remains, a driving force that is dynamically transforming the clinical and professional environment of nursing.[13–15] Thus, a high-level discussion and summary of the advantages, disadvantages, and implications for practice around how technology is impacting nursing is appropriate, and is the focus of the remainder of this article. The following topics—high reliability theory, big data, patient experience, patient care, and advocacy—organize this broad discussion.

HIGH RELIABILITY THEORY, TECHNOLOGY, AND NURSING

High reliability theory is based on the belief that accidents can be prevented through thoughtful organizational design that integrates accountability for safety at all organizational levels.[16] "High reliability organizations" (HROs) are those engaged in high-risk industries, such as aviation and nuclear power, which have developed standardized methods of practice to mitigate risk from human error. HROs incorporate an organizational commitment to safety with numerous system checks and balances, and strong organizational cultures for learning.[17] Because mistakes can cause serious consequences, including death, HROs are not afforded the opportunity of trial-and-error learning and, instead, rely on standardized processes and the critical thinking of all employees (**Box 1**).

The Institute of Medicine (IOM) report "To Err is Human" signaled the formal acknowledgment of how dangerously flawed the American health system is, and was followed by a second IOM report, "The Quality Chasm," which described how the American health care system could be redesigned to improve outcomes and decrease costs.[18,19]

> We live in a society absolutely dependent on science and technology and yet have cleverly arranged things so that almost no one understands science and technology. That's a clear prescription for disaster.
> —A quote from Carl Sagan, American Astrologer.

One response to the IOM reports has been for health care to recognize that it must become an HRO. Although an argument can be made that health care should not be compared with manufacturing cars or operating nuclear power plants, the frequency and severity of harm caused by the United States health care system compels adaptation of the characteristics of successful HROs.

Recent deployments of key technologies in health care are advancing the transformation toward high reliability.[20] The implementation of an EMR has been identified as a major tool for health care to become an HRO, and provides an excellent example of how technology can facilitate improvements in patient outcomes.[21] Although some health care organizations voluntarily adopted at least parts of an electronic record, it was not until the American Recovery and Reinvestment Act of 2009 made it mandatory that all health care providers demonstrate "meaningful use" of EMRs to maintain their existing Medicaid and Medicare reimbursement levels that full implementation of EMRs became widespread (**Fig. 1**).[22]

Before the EMR, the record of patient care was compiled in a paper chart that consisted of disparate sections for each discipline to handwrite their notes. It has been widely known that paper medical records are among the main contributing factors to medical errors made every day in health care facilities.[23] Recent literature has found

Box 1
Characteristics of High Reliability Organizations

Preoccupation with failure prevention and evaluation

Commitment to resilience and continuous improvement

Focus on operational systems failure rather than individual failure

A strong culture of safety

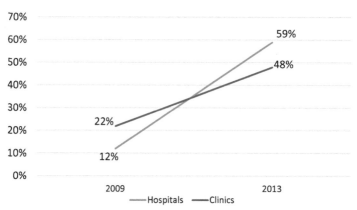

Fig. 1. Adoption of electronic medical records, 2009 through 2013. (*Adapted from* Pronovost PJ, Berenholtz SM, Goeschel CA, et al. Creating High Reliability in Health Care Organizations. Health Serv Res 2006;41:1599–617.)

that the presence of the EMR and other health information technology in the hospital setting has resulted in improved quality of nursing documentation.[24,25]

The EMR poses special challenges for nursing. The presence of the EMR and health information technology may cause several unintended consequences, such as over-dependence on technology and reduction in productivity while learning new technology. Additionally, end-users of an EMR may experience strong emotional responses as they struggle to adapt to new technology and disruptions in their workflow, especially those who lack computer skills.[26,27] Further, legal issues can arise from EMR documentation in the form of templates that may contain factually incorrect information or data that are beyond the scope of the author yet is authenticated by that author.[28] Privacy breaches are another grave concern in the age of the EMR, spanning from protected information left on an unattended computer screen to unauthorized access to medical records. Although technology can help nurses to provide safe care, it can also distract and consume valuable nurse/patient time. Nurses must learn to balance the benefits of new tools like the EMR with the impact on patients. Key to this balance is keeping the patient at the center of focus while using technology to strengthen the safety and quality of care provided.

BIG DATA, TECHNOLOGY, AND NURSING

In 2012, the IOM Committee on the Learning Health Care System released a report identifying the rising complexity of modern health care as 1 of 3 main areas that must be addressed to achieve better outcomes for patients. This report suggested that more effective use of health information technology is one approach to help manage the massive amount of patient data that are generated and stored, by guiding nurses and physicians in the decisions they make about patient care.[29]

> *Getting information off the internet is like drinking from a fire hose.*
> — *Mitchell Kapor, pioneer in the personal computing industry.*

Techniques developed to manage, analyze, and translate the vast and expanding amount of patient data elements, also known as 'big data,' that are stored in the

EMR will provide the foundation for much of the improvements in clinical practice and patient care that are yet to come.[30]

Many professional groups and clinicians agree that maintaining an evidence-based practice is the correct approach to most effectively and optimally approach decisions in patient care.[31,32] However, given the incredible volume of research and evidence that is generated each year and the time constraints facing clinicians, there are questions around the ability of health professionals to stay current with the literature or to access best practice information at the point of care to guide clinical practice.[33] Further, the literature has long described limitations in the human capacity to make factual or evidence-based decisions over time when faced with complexity, in the form of multiple or increasing options to choose from.[34,35] It follows that the effective translation and application of the best practice, evidence, or guideline in health care presents a pressing challenge for clinicians and technology alike.

> *What is evidence-based nursing?An ongoing process by which evidence, nursing theory and the practitioners' clinical expertise are critically evaluated and considered, in conjunction with patient involvement, to provide delivery of optimum nursing care for the individual.*
> *—From Scott K, McSherry R. Evidence Based Nursing: clarifying the concepts for nurses in practice. J Clin Nurs 2009;18(8):1085–95.*

There is early evidence that suggests that technology can offer valuable solutions in identifying and managing gaps in clinical information via just-in-time access to electronic clinical guidelines, decision, and practice support tools that can be embedded in the EMR to guide practice.[36,37] However, it is important to note that there is a large gap between what researchers and health systems believe electronic health technologies can do and what has been proven.[38]

Although there may be questions around how to best apply new and developing virtual technology to evidence-based health care delivery, there is certainty that effective data management and analysis of the big data contained in EMRs will result in valuable information, and holds great potential to generate a new standard of evidence and source of knowledge. Recent actual and proposed developments in big data analytics within the EMR are increasingly making this possible.[39,40]

> *The future of evidence-based careHealthcare accelerator Rock Health is predicting big advances for startups and healthcare providers using personalized, predictive analytic tools. The use of predictive analytics, essentially looking at historic data to predict future developments to directly intervene in patient care, will only increase as data multiplies, the report argues. In 2012, the healthcare system had stored roughly 500 petabytes of patient data, the equivalent of 10 billion four-drawer file cabinets full of information. By 2020, the healthcare system is projected to store 50 times as much information, 25,000 petabytes, meaning machine intelligence will be essential to complement human intelligence to make sense of it all.*
> *—Darius Tahir, from "Tech startups aim to dig through flood of healthcare data." Modern Healthcare. October 27, 2014. http://www.modernhealthcare.com/article/20141027/blog/310279996.*

To date, large, multisite randomized controlled trials have not been a typical nursing pathway for generating primary data or knowledge. They are expensive, and there are frequent institutional barriers for nurses in their conduction. Translating the 'big data' in the EMR to knowledge represents a golden opportunity for nursing to work around the institutional barriers encountered with randomized controlled trials, while still producing robust, highly powered results to inform clinical practice.[41]

A number of early approaches to tapping big data in the EMR are described in the literature, and have great potential to generate a new standard of evidence.[42] Retrospective chart review and data mining have been revolutionized by trigger methodology and natural language processing software run through the EMR, which search for the quantitative or qualitative data that the user requests, respectively.[43,44] These EMR data mining techniques were designed initially to identify patient safety events and trends, but are evolving along with EMR capabilities and big data to allow for expanded application, and represent yet another vehicle to connect nursing with the data needed to both explore and advance the quality of nursing care.

With EMR-based data mining in place, the bedside nurse can simply set the parameters she is interested in evaluating. For example, a nurse can request the data mining tool to search for any incidence of blood glucose less than 40 mg/dL in a newborn nursery over the past 30 days. A focused chart review takes place, with the disposition used to evaluate if a recently instituted neonatal feeding policy was effective at limiting hypoglycemia. Thus, the bedside nurse could mine and interpret these data at the point of care. These EMR data mining techniques are also an example of how technology can give bedside nurses comprehensive data from which they can advocate for patient and nursing needs that might otherwise be too resource intensive to identify or gather. The benefits of evidence-based cohort data, delivered when and how it is needed, at the fingertips of the nurse are obvious. The voice of the bedside nurse is critical in understanding what data need to be translated to actionable information, and how this information should be communicated in the patient care setting.[45]

PATIENT EXPERIENCE, TECHNOLOGY, AND NURSING

The patient experience is another primary force driving change in health care, with technology rapidly evolving to support the new model of the patient as the health care consumer. Smartphones, ubiquitous appendages in our world, allow patients instantaneous and unlimited access to an abundance of health-related information. Patients are presenting to nurses more informed and connected than ever before. Patients are using technology to research disease, treatment, and medications, as well as to connect with others who share health care experiences.[46]

Patients are able to "shop" hospitals, using transparent data like US News and World Report Top Hospital rankings or the Leapfrog Group's letter grades, to choose their hospital. They can also access a hospital website to determine the services available to them as a patient. A patient may choose a hospital based on hospitality services, such as access to private rooms, on-demand food service, and email access to the care team. This all translates into a more informed and empowered patient population who presents to the nurse with preconceived expectations about the hospital stay and course of treatment.[47]

A major advantage that technology yields to the patient experience is the increased control a patient has over the clinical encounter. Technology can facilitate a number of empowering functions for the patient right from their hospital bed. Hospital television (TV) systems have evolved to be tools for learning, communication and comfort (**Table 1**). A patient may turn on the TV and be immediately directed to a video that outlines how they can partner with the health care team to achieve optimum outcomes. Often this includes informing patients of their rights, standards that should be fulfilled by health care staff during the care process, and who to contact if the standards are not met.

Table 1
Not just a TV anymore: examples of offerings from an interactive patient care platform

Patient Experience	Health Education	Comfort Services
Access to health results (laboratory tests, diagnostic studies)	Admission orientation	On-demand movies and TV
Nurse call	Medication teaching	On-demand food services
Immediate feedback to department leaders	Diagnosis and treatment teaching	Games
Links to internal and external resources	Health promotion (smoking cessation, diet, and exercise)	Live broadcasts of activities (bingo, lecture series, etc.)
Virtual support groups	Discharge teaching with return demonstration and learning evaluation	Request housekeeping services

Technology that is used to support the patient experience can also have disadvantages. For example, many hospital systems have implemented immediate hand hygiene education for patients and families through their TV systems as part of the orientation to the hospital stay (**Fig. 2**; video link available at: http://www.cdc.gov/handhygiene/Patient_materials.html). The example of hand hygiene teaching through the TV system, although it is meant to empower the patient, can translate into a burden to some patients. Verbalizing concerns about lack of hand hygiene may be difficult, and the expectation that a patient will speak up may increase concern about the competency of the organization to provide safe care. Having the message come from the TV system rather than the traditional approach of the admitting nurse can establish a more depersonalized patient experience.

A depersonalized patient experience owing to integration of technology is increasingly becoming a concern. As technology becomes more integrated into the hospital

 Centers for Disease Control and Prevention
CDC 24/7: Saving Lives. Protecting People.™

Hand Hygiene Saves Lives: Patient Admission Video

This video, available in English and Spanish, teaches two key points to hospital patients and visitors to help prevent infections: the importance of practicing hand hygiene while in the hospital, and that it is appropriate to ask or remind their healthcare providers to practice hand hygiene as well.

Modeled after the video that airline passengers are required to view prior to take-off on a flight, this new video is intended to be shown to patients upon admission to the hospital. The goal is that the video will inform patients at the beginning of their hospital stay about what they can do to help prevent infections throughout the duration of their stay.

The video begins with a brief introduction on healthcare-associated infections. It is narrated by a nurse character named Gayle who stresses the importance of hand hygiene for both patients as well as healthcare providers.

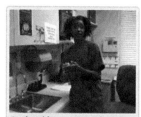
In the video, a nurse character named Gayle demonstrates hand hygiene using an alcohol-based hand sanitizer while emphasizing the importance of this practice to patients.

Fig. 2. A CDC video used to educate patients and families upon admission to the hospital. (*Courtesy of* the Centers for Disease Control and Protection.)

stay and bedside care, patients may feel less connected to their health care providers.[48]

> It's so critically important to recognize that hospitals and the people there provide more than clinical care. The "value" that a nurse or a tech provides to a patient is more than just administering medications or taking vitals. Value is often taking a moment to talk and make a patient feel comfortable upon admission.
>
> —Mark Graban, Lean blog 2010.

Technologically enhanced discharge teaching provides an example. Traditionally, preparing a patient for discharge and caring for themselves at home was accomplished through one-on-one teaching with the bedside nurse. However, many hospitals have found that the content and efficacy of these sessions are nurse dependent, and poor discharge teaching and preparation can lead to unanticipated readmissions. Recently, some hospitals have shifted to standard video-based discharge teaching.

This shift allows for flexibility for the patient to choose when they want to receive the teaching, because many are on demand, and allow patients and families to watch more than once if needed.[49] This flexibility is an advantage. However, this approach eliminates the interpersonal communication between the patient and the nurse. Lost is the connection, the face-to-face interaction, and the expression of care and concern that can be so meaningful to a patient anxious to go home with a new condition or treatment regimen.

The implications of the influence of technology on the patient experience are profound. Technology can be used to improve the efficiency of the care experience and can empower, teach, and connect the patient to the health care team. Technology can also depersonalize the care experience, reducing the frequency and quality of interpersonal interactions with the care team. Nurses must adapt to this chasm through understanding the effect technology can have on the patient experience and focusing on continuing to build strong relationships with patients. Through this approach, nurses can harness the positive power technology can have on the patient experience without allowing for the depersonalization of the patient experience.

PATIENT CARE, TECHNOLOGY, AND NURSING

The rise of technology is having significant impact for nurses at the bedside.[50] Technology is integrated in almost every task a nurse performs during a shift, from monitoring patient vital signs and performing assessments, to administering medications and documenting care (**Fig. 3**). According to the Agency for Healthcare Research and Quality, there are more than 5000 types of medical devices in use by health care providers.[51]

Technologic advances in health care are integrating human factor designs to help reduce human contributing errors during health care delivery. For example, intravenous medication administration pumps with smart technology can help to ensure a human error in programming does not result in a significant overmedication or undermedication of a dose to a patient.[52] Bar code medication administration, which is used to verify patient and medication accuracy, can assist the nurse validates and adheres to the 5 rights of medication administration (**Table 2**). These technologies support the nurse to provide safe care in an increasingly complex clinical environment.

Technology can contribute to a reduction of time to build the nurse–patient relationship, and it can also erode critical thinking skills key to effective nursing practice. In an

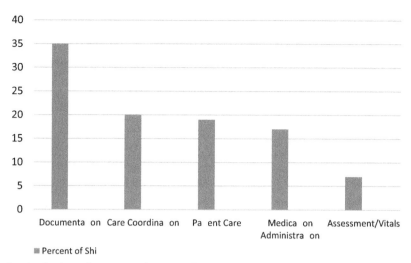

Fig. 3. Distribution of nursing tasks in a shift. (*Data from* Hendrich A, Chow MP, Skierczynski BA, et al. A 36-hospital time and motion study: how do medical-surgical nurses spend their time? Perm J 2008;12(3):30.)

effort to balance the tasks in a complex care environment, nurses may become reliant on the safeguarding technology.[53] A nurse may stop checking armbands before administering a medication, believing the technology to be error proof. Reports of medication errors owing to malfunctioning technology are common, with something as simple as a low battery on a medication scanner contributing to wrong patient administration when the nurse did not verify the system was functioning. As technology becomes more advanced, and is integrated into all aspects of care nurses provide, nurses must adapt while maintaining and advancing the skills at the heart of nursing.

The human spirit must prevail over technology.
—Albert Einstein.

ADVOCACY, TECHNOLOGY, AND NURSING

In 2011, the theoretic physicist Michio Kaku reminded a health care audience that a single smart phone holds more computing power than all of NASA had when they sent Neil Armstrong to the moon in 1969. Kaku also explained Moore's law, which (currently) assumes computing power will continue to double every 18–24 months.[54] With the current and anticipated accelerating pace of change in technological capacity, it is difficult to imagine what the relationship between technology and nursing will be like in 20 or even 30 years. Similarly uncertain is conversation around the relationship between nurses as advocates for patients in the age of advanced technology.

The techniques have galloped ahead of the concepts. We have moved away from studying the complexity of the organism; from processes and organization to composition
—Sir James Black, Nobel prize–winning pharmacologist, commenting on the growing use of new technologies.

Table 2
Examples of technology uses within 1 nursing task: Medication administration

Technology	Purpose
EHR via computer	Review MAR for medications ordered
Automated dispensing system—medication	Access medication
Automated dispensing system—supplies	Access medication administration supplies
Computer	Review medication profile via electronic pharmacology database
Bar code scanner	Verify correct patient and medication
IV pump	Facilitate medication administration
EHR via computer	Document the medication administration and patient's response to the medication

Abbreviations: EHR, electronic health record; IV, intravenous; MAR, medication administration record.

A recent example demonstrating how disruptive technology has been to the traditional relationship between the patient, provider, and health system is best described by the lived experience of Salvatore Iaconesi. He is an artist and open-source engineer from Italy who was diagnosed with brain cancer at age 39. Iaconesi rejected the way he was approached as a "disease on legs" by the medical system, and opened his clinical data up to the world on a website he named "La Cura."

> *When you have cancer you disappear. And you are replaced by someone/something else: a patient.*
> *—A quote by Salvatore Iaconesi, as part of an interview posted in the McGill Reporter, 2014.*

He invited anyone who could help him to find a cure to respond. He received more than 500,000 responses from around the world, weighed his options, applied many of the suggestions, and is now cancer free.[55] None of what Salvatore Iaconesi chose for himself would have been possible 25 years ago, and yet today his is just one of countless examples of how technology is redesigning the experience of health care.

The role of the nurse advocate for a patient like Iaconesi is not difficult to imagine. He sought and found a way to be treated holistically, which falls comfortably into the nursing model. However, how will nurses advocate for their 13 year old patient who tested positive for an autosomal-dominant and fatal disease through direct to consumer marketing for genetic testing? What exactly will be the role of the nurse as advocate for her patient who wants genetic engineering to ensure the intellectual quotient, sex, or eye color of their child? Or for the new baby who is the first recipient of a 3-dimensional printed heart?

These examples of future possibilities are proposed based on current realities. Given Moore's law, one must also consider the bulk of what is to come for technology and human health cannot even be imagined. Although bedside nurses cannot prepare for the unknown, they can and should be aware that patient care is now on a technological continuum that will likely be so changed as to be unrecognizable in 50 years. The nursing profession must begin to prepare itself now to move nimbly and rapidly forward with patients as their advocates, as technology continues the inexorable and often unpredictable transformation of the collective health care reality. For even in the virtual age, patients are adrift without the nurse who will recognize that technology is providing solutions, but that the right questions still need to be asked.

> *Computers are useless. They can only give you answers.*
> *—Pablo Picasso.*

SUMMARY

Changing how information is communicated to nurses, and how nurses communicate information, is a deceptively simple sounding concept. The successful translation of this concept to action, through patient centered technological interventions, is critical to the success of a redesigned health care system.[56] These changes, when weighed against the needs of patients and the demands of the health care system, seem inevitable. Nursing must prepare itself to guide and manage the changes in how health systems process, use and store patient data. Nurses must be involved in all steps of this redesign to ensure that the future course of technology in the patient care setting is guided by nurses, not for nurses.

REFERENCES

1. Hiestand WC. Think different: inventions and innovations by nurses, 1850 to 1950. Am J Nurs 2000;100(10):72–7.
2. Hiestand WC. Invisible inventors. A historical overview of creative midwives and nurses. Nurs Leadersh Forum 1999;4(1):18–25.
3. Sandelowski M. 'Making the best of things': technology in American nursing, 1870-1940. Nurs Hist Rev 1997;5:3–22.
4. Sandelowski M. Troubling distinctions: a semiotics of the nursing/technology relationship. Nurs Inq 1999;6:198–207.
5. Howell JD. Technology in the hospital: transforming patient care in the early twentieth century. Baltimore (MD): Johns Hopkins University Press; 1995.
6. Fukuyama F. Our posthuman future: consequences of the biotechnology revolution. New York: Farrar; 2002.
7. Facts about the nursing workforce. Available at: http://www.rwjf.org/en/research-publications/find-rwjf-research/2010/07/facts-about-the-nursing-workforce.html. Accessed November 22, 2014.
8. Kossman SP, Scheidenhelm SL. Nurses' perceptions of the impact of electronic health records on work and patient outcomes. Comput Inform Nurs 2008;26(2): 69–77.
9. Dahm MF, Wadensten B. Nurses' experiences of and opinions about using standardized care plans in electronic health records. Stud Health Technol Inform 2009;146:763–4.
10. Laramee A. Nurses' attitude toward the electronic health record still uncertain after 6 months. Heart Lung 2010;39(4):357–8.
11. Barnard A. A critical review of the belief that technology is a neutral object and nurses are its master. J Adv Nurs 1997;26(1):126–31.
12. Lu ZY, Chen WL, Chen HC, et al. Reflections on technology and nursing profession development. Hu Li Za Zhi 2009;56(3):88–92.
13. Axford RL, Carter BE. Impact of clinical information systems on nursing practice. Nurses' perspectives. Comput Nurs 1995;14(3):156–63.
14. Sandelowski M. Devices & desires: gender, technology, and American nursing. Chapel Hill (NC): University of North Carolina Press; 2000.

15. McNeil BJ, Elfrink VL, Bickford CJ, et al. Nursing information technology knowledge, skills, preparation of student nurses, nursing faculty, clinicians: a U.S. survey. J Nurs Educ 2003;42:341–9.

16. Sutcliffe KM. High Reliability Organizations (HROs). Best Practice & Research. Clinical Anesthesiology 2011;25(2):133–44.

17. Pronovost PJ, Berenholtz SM, Goeschel CA, et al. Creating high reliability in health care organizations. Health Serv Res 2006;41:1599–617.

18. Kohn LT, Corrigan JM, Donaldson MS, editors. To err is human: building a safer health system. Washington, DC: National Academy Press; 1999.

19. Institute of Medicine. Committee on quality health care in America. Crossing the quality chasm: a new health system for the 21st century. Washington, DC: National Academy Press; 2001.

20. Gaba DM. Structural and organizational issues in patient safety: a comparison of health care to other high-hazard industries. Calif Manage Rev 2000;43:83–102.

21. Chaudhry B, Wang J, Wu S, et al. Systematic review: impact of health information technology on quality, efficiency, and costs of medical care. Ann Intern Med 2006;144(10):742–52.

22. Jha AK, DesRoches CM, Campbell EG, et al. Use of electronic health records in U.S. hospitals. N Engl J Med 2009;360(16):1628–38.

23. Sullivan M. Playing catch-up in health care technology. J Health Care Compl 2010;12(3):25–30.

24. Waneka R, Spetz J. Hospital information technology systems' impact on nurses and nursing care. J Nurs Adm 2010;40(12):509–14.

25. Silow-Carroll S, Edwards JN, Rodin D. Using electronic health records to improve quality and efficiency: the experiences of leading hospitals. Issue Brief (Commonw Fund) 2012;17:1–38.

26. Menachemi N, Collum T. Benefits and drawbacks of electronic health record systems. Risk Manag Healthc Policy 2011;4:47–55.

27. Poissant L, Pereira J, Tamblyn R, et al. The impact of electronic health records on time efficiency of physicians and nurses: a systematic review. J Am Med Inform Assoc 2005;12(5):505–16.

28. Sittig D, Singh H. Legal, ethical, and financial dilemmas in electronic health record adoption and use. Pediatrics 2011;127(4):e1042–7.

29. Smith M, Saunders R, Stuckhardt L, et al. Best care at lower cost: the path to continuously learning health care in America. Washington, DC: The National Academies Press; 2012.

30. Murdoch TB, Detsky AS. The inevitable application of big data to health care. JAMA 2013;309(13):1351–2.

31. Geibert RC. Using diffusion of innovation concepts to enhance implementation of an electronic health record to support evidence-based practice. Nurs Adm Q 2006;30(3):203–10.

32. Piscotty R, Kalisch B. Nurses' use of clinical decision support: a literature review. Comput Inform Nurs 2014;32:562–8.

33. Del Fiol G, Workman T, Gorman PN. Clinical questions raised by clinicians at the point of care: a systematic review. JAMA Intern Med 2014;174(5):710–8.

34. Miller GA. The magical number seven, plus or minus two: some limits on our capacity for processing information. Psychol Rev 1956;63(2):81–97.

35. Cowan N. Metatheory of storage capacity limits. Behav Brain Sci 2001;24(1):154–76.

36. Kawamoto K, Houlihan CA, Balas EA, et al. Improving clinical practice using clinical decision support systems: a systematic review of trials to identify features critical to success. BMJ 2005;330:765.

37. Lobach D, Sanders GD, Bright TJ, et al. Enabling health care decision making through clinical decision support and knowledge management. Evidence report/technology assessment no. 203. Duke Evidence Based Practice Center. Rockville (MD): Agency for Healthcare Research and Quality; 2012. Report No.: 12-E001-EF.

38. Black AD, Car J, Pagliari C, et al. The impact of eHealth on the quality and safety of health care: a systematic overview. PLoS Med 2011;8:e1000387.

39. Stewart WF, Shah NR, Selna MJ, et al. Bridging the inferential gap: the electronic health record and clinical evidence. Health Aff 2007;26:181–91.

40. Hoffman S, Podgurski A. Improving health care outcomes through personalized comparisons of treatment effectiveness based on electronic health records. J Law Med Ethics 2011;39(3):425–36.

41. Dean BB, Lam J, Natoli JL, et al. Use of electronic medical records for health outcomes research: a literature review. Med Care Res Rev 2009;66(6):611–38.

42. Longhurst CA, Harrington RA, Shah NH. A 'green button' for using aggregate patient data at the point of care. Health Aff 2014;33(7):1229–35.

43. Resar RK, Rozich JD, Classen D. Methodology and rationale for the measurement of harm with trigger tools. Qual Saf Health Care 2003;12(Suppl 2):ii39–45.

44. Murff HJ, Patel VL, Hripcsak G, et al. Detecting adverse events for patient safety research: a review of current methodologies. J Biomed Inform 2003;36(1):131–43.

45. Park JI, Pruinelli L, Westra BL, et al. Applied nursing informatics research – state-of-the-art methodologies using electronic health record data. Stud Health Technol Inform 2014;201:395–400.

46. Or CK, Karsh BT. A systematic review of patient acceptance of consumer health information technology. J Am Med Inform Assoc 2009;16(4):550–60.

47. Barello S, Graffigna G, Vegni E. Patient engagement as an emerging challenge for healthcare services: mapping the literature. Nurs Res Pract 2012;2012:905934.

48. Barnard A, Sandelowski M. Technology and humane nursing care: (ir)reconcilable or invented difference? J Adv Nurs 2001;34(3):367–75.

49. Prey JE, Woollen J, Wilcox L, et al. Patient engagement in the inpatient setting: a systematic review. J Am Med Inform Assoc 2014;21:742–50.

50. Almerud S, Alapack RJ, Fridlund B, et al. Beleaguered by technology: care in technologically intense environments. Nurs Philos 2008;9(1):55–61.

51. ECRI Institute. Medical device safety reports. Available at: http://www.mdsr.ecri.org/default.aspx?v=1. Accessed November 30, 2014.

52. Rothschild JM, Keohane CA, Cook EF, et al. A controlled trial of smart infusion pumps to improve medication safety in critically ill patients. Crit Care Med 2005;33(3):533–40.

53. Ash JS, Berg M, Coiera E. Some unintended consequences of information technology in health care: the nature of patient care information system-related errors. J Am Med Inform Assoc 2004;11(2):104–12.

54. Buntz B. Theoretical physicist Michio Kaku predicts the future of healthcare. 2011. Available at: http://www.mddionline.com/article/theoretical-physicist-michio-kaku-predicts-future-healthcare. Accessed November 22, 2014.

55. Iaconesi S. My open source cure. My Open Source Cure. N.p., n.d. Web. 15 Nov. 2014. Available at: http://opensourcecureforcancer.com/. Accessed November 1, 2014.

56. Committee on the Robert Wood Johnson Foundation Initiative on the Future of Nursing, at the Institute of Medicine. The future of nursing: leading change, advancing health. Washington, DC: National Academies Press; 2011.

Blood Pressure and the Obese

Mindy McCallum Mullins, CRNA, DNAP

KEYWORDS

- Obesity • Blood pressure • Forearm • Oscillometric • Technology in operating room

KEY POINTS

- Although technological advancements may enhance patient care delivery, health care providers must question why and how specific tasks are performed, such as blood pressure measurement.
- A single abnormal blood pressure value may not dictate a treatment change. An inaccurately obtained measurement, however, may result in misdiagnosis and under- or overtreatment.
- Accuracy of blood pressure measurement in patients who are obese is contingent on many factors, including selection of proper cuff size and shape, location of measurement, and extremity characteristics. Measurement site circumference must be determined prior to cuff selection.
- Manufacturers of oscillometric monitoring devices either do not recommend forearm blood pressure measurements or do not provide valid, detailed, or reliable directions for obtaining measurements from the forearm.
- In the presence of numerous comorbidities or complex positioning with improper noninvasive blood pressure measurement technique, perioperative invasive blood pressure monitoring should be considered in patients who are obese to avoid harmful complications.

VALIDITY OF A FOREARM APPROACH IN OBTAINING PERIOPERATIVE BLOOD PRESSURE MEASUREMENTS IN PATIENTS WHO ARE OBESE

The worldwide prevalence of obesity has increased 60% since the year 2000 with the number of overweight individuals rivaling the number of underweight.[1,2] The World Health Organization estimates that by 2015 more than 2 billion individuals will be overweight, and of them 700 million will be obese.[2] Individuals classified as obese have a body weight greater than 30% above ideal body weight and a body mass index (BMI) equal to or greater than 30 kg/m².[3]

Disclosure: None.
Department of Anesthesia, Baptist Memorial Hospital North Mississippi, 2301 South Lamar Boulevard, Oxford, MS 38655, USA
E-mail address: mmullins45@yahoo.com

Nurs Clin N Am 50 (2015) 241–255
http://dx.doi.org/10.1016/j.cnur.2015.03.009   nursing.theclinics.com
0029-6465/15/$ – see front matter © 2015 Elsevier Inc. All rights reserved.

With the prevalence of obesity escalating globally, an increasing number of patients who are obese are seeking elective or requiring emergency surgery. Certified registered nurse anesthetists (CRNAs) are challenged daily to provide vigilant, safe care. New technology, equipment integrity, and patient positioning are a constant concern as are CRNAs' dependence on technological devices to monitor physiologic variables, such as oxygen saturation, carbon dioxide level, blood pressure measurement, and electrocardiogram. Effective hemodynamic monitoring guides the administration of anesthesia and enables the CRNA to recognize patient deterioration prior to irreversible and detrimental complications. The ability to provide supportive therapy and make anesthetic adjustments is often hindered with obesity, especially in relation to ineffective blood pressure monitoring.

Studies dating from 1954 have investigated the validity and reliability of blood pressure monitoring techniques in individuals who are obese.[4,5] The validity of blood pressure measurements obtained with a cuff are often questioned, and the use of an arterial catheter for invasive blood pressure monitoring is associated with potential risks, such as infection and trauma. Additionally, invasive monitoring is often impractical and difficult to place in patients who are obese.

In the clinical setting, CRNAs routinely obtain blood pressure measurements from the forearm of patients who are obese. The primary reason for the alternative approach is poor cuff size fitting in relation to the upper arm's circumference, conical shape, and length. Current recommendations concerning the optimal location of a blood pressure cuff for forearm measurement have yet to be established. The purpose of this project was to explore evidence-based literature to determine the validity of a forearm approach in obtaining perioperative blood pressure measurements in patients who are obese.

SIGNIFICANCE OF THE PROBLEM
Society in General

Obesity ranks as the fifth leading cause of global deaths and surpasses tobacco as the leading cause of preventable death.[2] Obesity is more prevalent in men than women, and individuals with a BMI greater than 30 kg/m^2 have a decreased life expectancy of 2 to 4 years in comparison with healthier individuals.[6] Individuals classified as morbidly obese, with a BMI greater than 40 kg/m^2, have an additional reduction of 8 to 10 years.[6] More than 300,000 American adults die annually of causes directly associated with obesity.[7]

The obesity epidemic is not limited to the adult population. Internationally, 42 million children under the age of 5 are overweight, and epidemiologists predict that children's lives will be shorter than their parents'.[2,8,9] Childhood obesity has been linked to low socioeconomic status, low education levels, high unemployment rates, and high-calorie food.[10,11] The prevalence of childhood and adolescent obesity represents a major health concern toward the susceptibility of acquiring noncommunicable diseases at an earlier age.[12] Public health advocates, health care industries, and government officials have yet to identify a compelling way of reversing obesity in today's youth.[12]

Obesity poses a challenge for the nation's overall economy by having an impact on public health and productivity.[9] The national estimated cost of obesity exceeds $254 billion annually.[10] The principal cause of employee absenteeism is health issues attributed to obesity, with lost productivity reported to be more than $153 billion annually.[9] The Congressional Budget Office anticipates that obesity related spending will escalate another 60% by 2020.[8]

Health Care

Obesity has become a significant health concern in the United States.[13] Health care spending related to obesity was $147 billion in 2008; 21% of total national health care spending.[9] Hospitals are remodeling facilities to accommodate individuals who are obese, including enlarging doorways and equipment, and billions of dollars are spent annually for obesity-related illnesses.[14] Health policy experts O'Grady and Capretta[9] project that medical costs related to the obesity epidemic could exceed $861 billion by 2030.

Although disagreement exists about whether obesity is an independent risk factor for increased morbidity and mortality perioperatively, several studies conclude that obesity is an independent predictor of late mortality.[15–17] In a landmark study, Bamgbade[18] analyzed postoperative complications in 6773 patients treated at the University of Michigan between 2001 and 2005. The findings establish that patients who are obese have higher rates of postoperative complications that include 5 times more myocardial infarctions and 4 times more peripheral nerve injuries.[18] In addition, the death rate among patients classified as morbidly obese was twice as high.[18]

Bariatric surgery is among the most cost-effective interventions to improve the health status of individuals who are obese.[9,19] Bariatric surgical procedures are performed to facilitate weight loss and account for approximately 113,000 cases annually with associated costs of $1.5 billion.[20] As the number of individuals seeking bariatric surgery increases worldwide, the physiologic and mechanical changes of obesity must be considered by CRNAs to ensure clinically effective and safe care that reduces morbidity, mortality, hospital stay, and cost.[21]

Clinical Nurse Anesthesia Practice

Obesity-related comorbidities that are associated with metabolic disease and mechanical impairment create considerable challenges for CRNAs.[7,18,21,22] The presence and severity of comorbidities may be concealed by a sedentary lifestyle and emerge during the perioperative period.[22] Perioperatively, CRNAs use blood pressure measurements to assess a patient's cardiovascular status and response to anesthetic agents, clinical conditions, intravenous fluids, medications, positioning, and surgical stimulation. Many anesthetic drugs, inhaled and injectable, cause blood vessel dilation and depress heart function.[7] With the effects of age, disease process, and surgical procedures, the vascular system and heart may be further compromised resulting in decreased profusion of vital organs, such as the brain and kidneys.[21] If insufficient blood flow is available to meet an organ's metabolic needs, irreversible damage may occur, and, on rare occurrences, death may result.[18]

Abnormal blood pressure measurements prompt CRNAs to repeat measurements and further investigate potential causes of blood pressure variances. Although a single abnormal value may not dictate a treatment change, an inaccurately obtained blood pressure measurement may result in misdiagnosis and under- or overtreatment. Accuracy of blood pressure measurement in patients who are obese is contingent on many factors, including selection of proper cuff size and shape, location of measurement, and extremity characteristics.[5] Vigilant hemodynamic monitoring and treatment of symptoms associated with comorbidities are essential in preventing perioperative complications and obtaining a safe anesthetic outcome for patients who are obese.[21]

CONCEPTUAL FRAMEWORK FOR PROJECT

As the prevalence of obesity increases, CRNAs caring for patients who are obese across the lifespan are faced with unique demands in all practice settings. Even basic assessment techniques, such as effective noninvasive blood pressure measurement, present numerous obstacles centered on the selection of the proper size cuff and placement. The conceptual model that guided this project (Capstone project) depicts concepts associated with blood pressure measurement and the interrelationships between the concepts when obtaining valid noninvasive measurements in patients who are obese perioperatively (**Boxes 1** and **2, Fig. 1**).

Blood Pressure Physiology

Blood pressure represents the hydrostatic force exerted by circulating blood against the inner walls of the arterial blood vessels in the vascular system.[26,27] The system consists of the heart, blood, and blood vessels and functions as a conduit for circulating blood. The 3 major types of vessels constituting the system include the arteries that transport oxygenated blood away from the heart; the capillaries that allow the exchange of chemicals, gases, and fluids between the blood and the tissues; and the veins that transport deoxygenated blood from the capillaries back toward the heart.[26]

Although the force occurs throughout the vascular system, the term, *blood pressure*, refers to the pressure within the arteries that are supplied by branches of the aorta.[27] Arterial blood pressure increases and decreases in a pattern analogous with the cardiac cycle.[26] The pressure is dependent on the heart's pumping pressure, the arterial wall's resistance, the elasticity of the blood vessels, the circulating blood volume, and the blood's viscosity.[26,27] Numerous forces are involved with the movement of blood throughout the system, which include hydrostatic pressure, gravity, kinetic and potential energy provided by the cardiac pump, and pressure gradients (differences between any 2 points).[26,27] During ventricular contraction, blood is expressed out and into the pulmonary trunk and aorta, significantly increasing the pressure within the arteries. The maximal aortic pressure succeeding ventricular ejection signifies the systolic pressure.[26,27] After ejection, the left ventricle relaxes and refills, and the pressure within the aorta falls.[26,27] The lowest pressure remaining in the arteries prior to ventricular ejection signifies diastolic pressure.[26,27]

The standard reference for measuring blood pressure is the mercury manometer; therefore, blood pressure is stated in mm Hg.[26] In the adult arterial system, the systolic pressure averages 120 mm Hg, and the diastolic pressure averages 80 mm Hg.[28] Classifications of blood pressure measurement values according to the American Heart Association (AHA) are depicted in **Table 2**.[29]

Methods of Blood Pressure Measurement

Blood pressure measurement can be obtained indirectly by cuff devices or directly by arterial cannulation and pressure transduction. Indirect blood pressure measurement methods consist of manual intermittent technique (auscultatory) or automated intermittent technique (oscillometric). The auscultatory method is considered the gold standard of noninvasive blood pressure measurement.[30] Direct blood pressure

---

Box 1
Body mass index

Adolphe Quetelet, a Belgian mathematician and statistician, devised a simple index for classifying human body shape relative to ideal body weight for height.[23] The BMI, or Quetelet index, is calculated as weight in kilograms divided by height in meters squared (kg/m^2).[23] BMI values are age-independent and identical for both men and women.[23] The index is used to classify underweight, normal weight, overweight, or obesity.

<table>
<tr><td>

Box 2
Obesity classification

The obesity classification estimates relative risk of morbidity and mortality in comparison to ideal body weight. The cutoff points are established to determine the level of overweight or obesity in adult men and adult nonpregnant women from all racial and ethnical groups.[24] According to the World Health Organization, an individual with a BMI of greater than 30 kg/m^2 is classified as obese **(Table 1)**.[24,25]

</td></tr>
</table>

measurement consists of percutaneous radial artery cannulation or an alternative arterial pressure monitoring site.

In 1876, Étienne-Jules Marey first demonstrated the oscillometric technique.[31] During oscillometric blood pressure measurement, a sphygmomanometer cuff with a pressure sensor is used to indicate the pulsation of the artery wall as a pressure vibration or oscillation, which is interpreted as the blood pressure value.[30] The cuff is inflated beyond the point at which vibrations or oscillations cease and slowly deflated.[30] A sensor within the cuff recognizes the first vibration and interprets that as the systolic pressure value, the mean arterial pressure corresponds to larger vibrations, and the diastolic value is interpreted from the last vibration.[30] The cuff automatically deflates in increments of 5 to 10 mm Hg.[30] The technology of oscillation interpretation is specific for each manufacturer.[30] The accuracy of the oscillation pattern's recording depends on the anatomic position, elasticity and size of the artery, and the distribution of surrounding tissues.[30]

Invasive blood pressure monitoring, considered the gold standard among all blood pressure measurement methods, provides continuous, real-time blood pressure values numerically and graphically.[30] The technique involves direct measurement of arterial pressure by placement of a cannula needle in an artery (radial, brachial, axillary, femoral, or dorsalis pedis). After insertion, the cannula is attached to a fluid-filled, sterile system that transmits pressure waves to an externally mounted transducer.

Measurement Site Circumference, Shape, and Length

To avoid inaccurate blood pressure measurements, measurement site circumference must be determined prior to cuff selection.[32] Circumference of an object is defined as the linear distance around the edge of a spherical object at the largest part. For example, upper arm circumference is determined by measuring midway between the olecranon and the acromion process in centimeters.[32]

Bonso and colleagues[32] discovered that the shape of the upper arm is troncoconical in virtually all individuals; the difference between the proximal and the distal upper arm ranges from 1 to 20 cm, and arm shapes vary according to circumference,

Table 1
1997 World Health Organization obesity classification

Classification	Body Mass Index (kg/m^2)
Underweight	<18.50
Normal weight	18.50–24.99
Overweight	>25.00
Obese	≥30.00
Morbid obesity	≥40.00

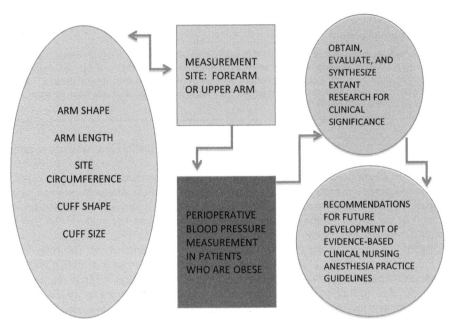

Fig. 1. Conceptual framework guiding project.

gender, and obesity classification. With all anthropometric variables included, arm circumference causes the most variances in the conicity index.[32] In patients who are morbidly obese, very large arm circumferences in the presence of short humeral length result in cuff extension past the elbow by several centimeters, creating inaccurate blood pressure measurements.[32–34]

Blood Pressure Cuff Shape

Patients who are obese commonly have short, conical shaped upper arms with large circumferences, making correct placement and filling of blood pressure cuffs difficult.[33] Three distinct shapes delineate measurement location and cuff shape, which include cylindrical, cone, and truncated cone.[34] A cylindrical object is defined as a 3-D object bounded by a curved surface with 2 parallel circles of equal size at the ends. In comparison, a cone object tapers from a circular section to a point. Truncated cones are described as cutting a cone between 2 parallel planes, thereby shortening the length.

Table 2
2013 American Heart Association blood pressure categories

Blood Pressure Category	Systolic (mm Hg)	Diastolic (mm Hg)
Normal	<120	<80
Prehypertension	120–139	80–89
Hypertension (stage 1)	140–159	90–99
Hypertension (stage 2)	≥160	≥100
Hypertensive crisis	>180	>110

Blood Pressure Cuff Size

Miscuffing constitutes the most frequent blood pressure measurement error, with under-cuffing accounting for 84% of miscuffing in large arms.[34,35] The proper cuff size relative to measurement location circumference is crucial for obtaining a valid blood pressure measurement.[35] Blood pressure cuffs that are too large yield measurements lower than actual values, whereas blood pressure cuffs that are too small yield measurements higher than actual values.[34,35] According to the AHA, the ideal blood pressure cuff size should have a bladder length of 80% of the site's circumference, a width that is 40% of the site's circumference, and a length to width ratio of 2:1.[36] **Table 3** outlines the AHA's cuff size recommendations.[36]

Location of Measurement

The standard location for blood pressure measurement is the brachial artery in the upper arm (area from the shoulder to the elbow) with the arm positioned at heart level (level of the right atrium).[35–37] The forearm (area from the elbow to the wrist) is often used as an alternative site of blood pressure measurement when available cuffs do not fit a patient's upper arm or the upper arm is inaccessible.[37] Additional sites where blood pressure measurement are obtained include calf, finger, thigh, and wrist.[35,36]

Blood pressure measurements are influenced by the arm's position.[35,38] The pressure progressively increases approximately 5 to 6 mm Hg as the arm moves from horizontal to vertical position, which is expected with hydrostatic pressure changes.[35] Systolic and diastolic pressures differ substantially in distinct parts of the arterial tree with systolic pressure increasing and diastolic pressure decreasing in more distal arteries.[35] The decrease in pressure along any segment of the arterial system is due to resistance and conversion of potential into kinetic energy. The pressure decrease as a result of energy lost in overcoming resistance is irreversible, because energy is dissipated as heat.[39] The pressure decrease due to conversion of potential into kinetic energy as narrowing of the vessel occurs is reversed when the vessel widens once again.[39]

Two physics principles may explain discrepancies of blood pressure measurements obtained in various locations, especially upper arm and forearm. When blood steadily flows from one point in the vascular system to another, the volume's total energy content along any given streamline remains constant, providing no frictional losses.[39] According to the Bernoulli principle, as flow velocity increases in a vessel, lateral pressure distending the vessel walls decreases.[39] Pressure falls slightly in medium- and large-sized arteries because resistance to flow is low, but pressure falls rapidly in smaller arteries and arterioles, which are the primary sites of peripheral resistance against which the heart pumps.[39] Poiseuille law predicts the volume of flow under laminar flow conditions in straight tubes or vessels where wall friction is not a significant factor.[39] As the diameter of a vessel increases, flow increases, and as the diameter of a vessel decreases, flow decreases.[39]

Table 3
2005 American Heart Association cuff size recommendations

Cuff	Arm Circumference (cm)	Bladder Width (cm)	Bladder Length (cm)
Small adult	22–26	10	24
Adult	27–34	13	30
Large adult	35–44	16	38
Adult thigh	45–52	20	42

LITERATURE ANALYSIS

Critical analysis of existing evidence investigating the relationship between the fore-arm and upper arm approaches in obtaining blood pressure measurements in patients who are obese is challenging because of

- Use of different blood pressure measurement techniques (arm and cuff placement in relation to a participant's heart level, precise body position of the participant at the time of measurement, cuff size in accordance to arm circumference, timing of sequential measurements, and number of consecutive measurements at one site)
- Inconsistent measurement devices, and
- Variations in investigators' attention to conceptual definitions

Information regarding participants' demographic (age, race, and gender) information, anthropometric (arm circumference, BMI, and skinfold measurement) dimensions, and clinical diagnoses varies among studies. In a majority of studies, recruiting young healthy adults and eliminating individual characteristics that might influence blood pressure measurements, such as known cardiac arrhythmias or unstable medical condition, controlled sample selection.[40–44]

Pierin and colleagues,[42] Vinyoles and colleagues,[45] Schell and colleagues,[43,44,46,47] Domiano and colleagues,[48] and Leblanc and colleagues[49] reported participants classified as obese as defined by a BMI greater than 30 kg/m^2; however, only 1 study[49] reported participants classified as morbidly obese separately. In 2 studies[42,49] in which obesity was required for inclusion in the sample, comparison of the conclusions with individuals who are classified as normal weight is not attainable. Numerous studies included participant arm circumference.[42,43,46–51] Trout and colleagues[52] and Schell and colleagues[47] explored the role of tissue composition in blood pressure measurement. Domiano and colleagues[48] and Schell and colleagues[47] evaluated the relationship between participant demographics and the difference in upper arm and forearm blood pressure measurements. Schell and colleagues[47] enhanced the investigation by additionally evaluating the influence of participants' demographics, anthropometrics, clinical diagnoses, and medications on upper arm and forearm blood pressure measurement differences.

Individual and Aggregate Findings

In the studies reviewed, 4 studies[40,51–53] used the auscultatory method for obtaining blood pressure measurements noninvasively, whereas the remaining studies[41–50,54] used the oscillometric method for obtaining blood pressure measurements that is the method predominately used today.

Across studies, a convenience sampling technique was used, and a majority of studies recruited young healthy adults and eliminated individual characteristics that might influence blood pressure measurements, such as known cardiac arrhythmias or unstable medical condition.[40–44] Nonprobability sampling technique is used when investigators consider the testing to be so basic and universal that the findings can be generalized beyond such a narrow sample. The generalizability of findings to complex positions (Trendelenburg, reverse Trendelenburg, prone, lateral, and lithotomy) may be limited because a majority of participants were seated or supine when blood pressure measurements where obtained.[40–45,48–54] In addition, the exact location of the upper arm and forearm was not disclosed in numerous studies.[40,42,45,50–53]

Five studies'[42,45,49,52,53] primary objective was to ascertain the influence of obesity in obtaining valid blood pressure measurements, whereas 2 studies[43,52] explored the effects of anatomic structures in obtaining valid blood pressure measurements. Of the studies including participants classified as obese, most studies[42–48] discovered that adults who are obese have the greatest difference between upper arm and forearm blood pressure measurements, making diagnosis and treatment of cardiac instability complex. Five studies[44,46,47,49,54] used Bland-Altman analysis to determine agreement between upper arm and forearm blood pressure measurements of systolic, diastolic, and mean arterial pressures. The Bland-Altman analysis is considered a more relevant analysis when measurements of individual participants are examined as well as determining if a new method can replace an old method or if the 2 methods can be interchangeable.[55]

Numerous studies[56–58] validating the accuracy of specific manufacturers' models of noninvasive oscillometric devices have been conducted. The International Organization for Standardization (ISO) 81060-2:2009 (mean difference ±5 mm Hg, with SD ≤8 mm Hg) is the standard used by the Association of the Advancement of Medical Instrumentation and manufacturers of oscillometric devices to test devices against mercury sphygmomanometers.[59] Devices adhering to the regulation are often used in health care settings.[59] The accuracy of oscillometric devices is validated for blood pressure measurements in the upper arm only, thus decreasing the validity of the findings.[59–61] The findings of the studies[41–50,54] revealed discrepancies between forearm and upper arm blood pressure measurements without reporting in accordance with ISO 81060-2:2009, thus introducing the risk of measurement error.

Strengths and Limitations

Numerous sources of potential errors exist in extant research that include failure of the investigators to use consistent measurement devices, define cuff placement in relation to the heart, describe the precise arm and body positions of the participants, and describe the methods used to measure blood pressures resulting in discrepancies and inconsistent findings.[62] Despite inconsistent monitoring devices and measurement methods, a majority of extant evidence[40,42–48,50,52–54] discourages a forearm approach as an alternative to an upper arm approach in obtaining noninvasive oscillometric blood pressure measurements. In addition, manufacturers of oscillometric monitoring devices used in health care settings today either do not recommend forearm blood pressure measurements or do not provide valid, detailed, or reliable directions for obtaining measurements from the forearm.[60,61] The quality of existing evidence strongly warrants further investigation of the forearm approach in obtaining valid blood pressure measurements in patients who are obese with unified blood pressure measurement methods, data collection procedures, and inclusion and exclusion criteria.

ETHICAL CONSIDERATIONS

Automated oscillometric blood pressure measurement devices have replaced the sphygmomanometer and stethoscope when noninvasively monitoring a patient's cardiovascular status and depth of anesthesia perioperatively. Although blood pressure monitoring devices are validated by manufacturers prior to consumer use, sources of human error related to cuff size and placement remain. In medical device validation studies, newly developed devices are compared with previously validated devices in nonrandomized, small populations with the use of a placebo often considered unethical.[63] Medical devices are separated into 3 classes, with class I minimal risk, class II intermediate risk, and class III substantial risk.[63] Oscillometric blood pressure cuffs pose minimal risks to human participants; therefore, the device is considered class I with no clinical trial requirement.[63] Regardless of class, the regulatory stipulations of medical device studies are the same, which include financial disclosure, informed consent, and institutional review board requirements.[63,64]

Regarding the nurse's role in promoting ethical practice in every setting, the American Nurses Association (ANA) states, "nurses are obligated to provide fair and equal treatment that respects the inherent worth, dignity, and uniqueness of every individual, unrestricted by considerations of social or economic status, personal attributes, or nature of the health problem."[65] The Code of Ethics for Nurses[65] also addresses the nurse's responsibility and accountability for individual nursing practice, which includes respect for autonomy, beneficence, nonmaleficence, and justice. Inadvertent discrimination, a violation of human rights, exists when invalidated methods of patient monitoring are used to obtain noninvasive blood pressure measurements from patients who are obese. Furthermore, practice settings are strengthened when nurses refuse to practice in a manner that has a negative impact on quality of care, patient safety, and clinical outcomes.[65] The ANA Code of Ethics for Nurses[65] and the American Association of Nurse Anesthetists (AANA) Standards of Nurse Anesthesia Practice[66] professionally and ethically bind CRNAs to provide evidence-based, high-quality patient care to all individuals regardless of circumstance and practice setting.

EVIDENCE-BASED RECOMMENDATIONS

Decades after the forearm approach was proposed in an effort to solve problems related to inadequate cuff size in relation to large arms, extant research does not provide a clear understanding of the difficulties associated with the use of the forearm in obtaining valid blood pressure measurements. Physiologic and anatomic explanations exist accounting for the differences between upper arm and forearm blood pressure measurements.[26,27,67] Fonseca-Reyes and colleagues[68] report that for each 5 cm increase in arm diameter, both systolic and diastolic blood pressure measurements are overestimated by 1 to 5 mm Hg; additionally, the forearm routinely yields elevated measurements in comparison to the upper arm (reported variances of 2.3–33 mm Hg).[40–52,54,68] Numerous factors also influence blood pressure measurement, such as sympathetic nervous system stimulation, positioning, age, genetics, comorbidities, and medications, which all emerge during the perioperative period.[7,18,21,22,69]

Validation of a forearm approach is clinically relevant considering the limitations related to perioperative blood pressure assessment methods in patients who are obese. The CRNA should be diligent in every attempt to obtain perioperative blood pressure measurements from the upper arm by ensuring that various cuff shapes and sizes are readily available. Consequently, the AHA declares that if the appropriate cuff shape or size is not available, blood pressure measurements could be obtained from the forearm according to the following recommendation: selecting appropriate cuff size as established by the AHA (see **Table 3**), auscultating the radial artery, placing oscillometric cuff with hoses exiting cuff over the radial artery, positioning the forearm at heart level, and documenting site of measurement.[28,29] Health care providers should be aware that systolic, diastolic, and mean blood pressure measurement values vary appreciably in the upper arm and forearm, and clinically acceptable discrepancies should be decided prior to measurement.[28,29]

Considering the findings of extant research and invalidation of oscillometric monitoring devices in accordance with the ISO 81060-2:2009 regulation, CRNAs have both the professional and ethical obligation to provide evidence-based, high-quality care as established by the AANA Standards of Nurse Anesthesia Practice guidelines and the ANA Code of Ethics for Nurses.[40,42–48,50,52–54,59,65,66] In the presence of numerous comorbidities or complex positioning with improper noninvasive blood pressure measurement technique, perioperative invasive blood pressure monitoring should be considered in patients who are obese to avoid harmful complications.[30,69-72] Furthermore, because of the lack of detailed and reliable information on blood pressure assessment in the forearm from experts and manufacturers of oscillometric monitoring devices, further investigation of the validity of the technique and development of an evidence-based clinical nursing anesthesia practice guideline is warranted.[36,40,42-51,54,59-61]

ACKNOWLEDGMENTS

The author gratefully acknowledges the support and guidance of Dr Katrin Sames, Chair, Professor, Middle Tennessee School of Anesthesia; and Drs Michael Vollman and Rachel Brown, Committee Members, Professors, Middle Tennessee School of Anesthesia.

REFERENCES

1. World Watch Institute. Chronic hunger and obesity epidemic; eroding global progress. Available at: http://www.worldwatch.org/press/news/200/03/04/. Accessed February 14, 2014.
2. World Health Organization (WHO). Obesity and overweight. Fact sheet N311. Available at: http://who.int. Accessed February 14, 2014.
3. Ogden CL, Carroll MD, Kit BK, et al. Prevalence of obesity in the United States, 2009–2010. NCHS Data Brief 2012;82:1–8.
4. Ven Bergen FH, Buckely JJ, French LA. Comparison of indirect and direct methods of measuring arterial blood pressure. Circulation 1954;10:481–90.
5. King GE. Errors in clinical measurement of blood pressure in obesity. Clin Sci 1967;32:223.
6. American Heart Association. With a very heavy heart. Obesity and cardiovascular disease. Available at: http://www.heart.org/idc/groups/heart-public/@wcm/@adv/documents/downloadable/ucm_428447.pdf. Accessed September 23, 2013.
7. Dindo D, Muller MK, Weber M, et al. Obesity in general elective surgery. Lancet 2003;361:2032–5.
8. Kaplan L. Obesity: the economic case in action. The Hill's Congress Blog. Available at: http://thehill.com/blogs/congress-blog/healthcare/217579-obesity-the-economic-case-for-action. Accessed September 29, 2013.
9. O'Grady MJ, Capretta JC. Assessing the economics of obesity and obesity interventions. Campaign to End Obesity. Available at: http://ogradyhp.com/yahoo_site_admin/assets/docs/Obesity_Paper_3-15-12_OGrady__Capretta.8282606.pdf. Accessed September 29, 2013.
10. Go AS, Mozaffarian D, Roger VL, et al. On behalf of the American Heart Association Statistics Committee and Stroke Statistics Subcommittee. Heart disease and stroke statistics 2013 update: a report from the American Heart Association. Circulation 2013;127:e6–245. Available at: http://www.heart.org/policyfactsheets. Accessed September 22, 2013.
11. Ogden C, Carroll M. Prevalence of obesity among children and adolescents: United States, trends 1963–1965 through 2007–2008. NCHS Health E-Stat. Available at: http://www.cdc.gov/nchs/data/hestat/obesity_child_07_08/obesity.pdf. Accessed October 1, 2013.
12. Kersh R, Stroup D, Taylor W. Childhood obesity: a framework for policy approaches and ethical consideration. Prev Chronic Dis 2011;8(5):A93. Available at: http://cdc.gov/pcd/issues/2011/sep10_0273.htm. Accessed October 1, 2013.

13. McTigue KM, Harris R, Hemphill B, et al. Screening and interventions for obesity in adults: summary of the evidence for the U.S. preventive services task force. Ann Intern Med 2003;139(11):933–49.

14. Massachusetts General Hospital. Supersize hospitals: by widening doorways and buying bariatric equipment, hospitals are adapting to a growing populous. Pronto. Massachusetts General Hospital. 2002. Available at: www.massgeneral.org. Accessed February 14, 2014.

15. National Institute of Health and Clinical Excellence. Obesity: the prevention, identification, assessment and management of overweight and obesity in adults and children. 2006. Available at: www.nice.org.uk/guidance/CG43. Accessed March 15, 2014.

16. Arterbum D, Livingston EH, Schifftner T. Predictors of long-term mortality after bariatric surgery performed in Veterans Affairs medical centers. Arch Surg 2009;144(10):914–20.

17. Van Straten AH, Bramer S, Soliman Hamad MA. Effect of body mass index on early and late mortality after coronary artery bypass grafting. Ann Thorac Surg 2010;89(1):30–7.

18. Bamgbade OA. Postoperative complications in obese and nonobese patients. World J Surg 2007;31(3):556–60.

19. Begley CE, Lairson DR, Morgan RO, et al. Evaluating the healthcare system. Chicago: Health Administration Press; 2013.

20. Livingston EH. The incidence of bariatric surgery has plateaued in the U.S. Am J Surg 2009;200(3):378–85.

21. Flegal KM, Kit BK, Orphana H. Association of all-cause mortality with overweight and obesity using standard body mass index categories: a systematic review and meta-analysis. JAMA 2013;309(1):71–82.

22. Leykin V, Brodsky JB. Controversies in the anesthetic management of the obese surgical patient. New York: Springer; 2012.

23. Eknoyan G. Adolphe Quetelet (1796–1874)-the average man and indices of obesity. Nephrol Dial Transplant 2008;23(1):47–51.

24. World Health Organization. Global database on body mass index. BMI classification. 2006. Available at: http://apps.who.int/bmi/index.jsp?introPage=intro_3.html. Accessed December 6, 2013.

25. U.S. Department of Health and Human Services. National Institute of Health. Classification of overweight and obesity. National Heart, Lung, and Blood Institute. 1997. Available at: http://nhlbi.nih.gov/guidelines/obesity/e_txtbk/txgd/414.htm. Accessed December 6, 2013.

26. Hall JE, Guyton AC. Textbook of medical physiology. Philadelphia: Saunders; 2006.

27. Shier D, Butler J, Lewis R. Hole's essentials of human anatomy and physiology. New York: McGraw-Hill Companies, Inc.; 2006.

28. U.S. Department of Health and Human Services. National Institutes of Health. The seventh report of the joint national committee on prevention, detection, evaluation, and treatment of high blood pressure (JNC 7). National Heart, Lung, and Blood Institute. 2013. Available at: http://www.nhlbi.nih.gov. Accessed December 1, 2013.

29. American Heart Association. Understanding blood pressure readings. 2013. Available at: www.heart.org/HEARTORG/Conditions/HighBloodPressure/. Accessed December 1, 2013.

30. Chu LF, Fuller AJ. Manual of clinical anesthesiology. Philadelphia: Lippincott Williams & Wilkins; 2011.

31. Stork M, Jilek J. Cuff pressure pulse waveforms: their current and prospective applications in biomedical instrumentation. In: Laskovski A, editor. Biomedical engineering trends in electronics, communications and software. InTech; 2011. Available at: http://www.intechopen.com/books/biomedical-engineering-trends-in-electronics-communications-andsoftware/cuff-pressure-pulse-waveforms-their-current-and-prospective-applications-in-biomedicalinstrumentati.

32. Bonso E, Saladini F, Zanier A, et al. Accuracy of a single rigid conical cuff with standard-sized bladder coupled to an automatic oscillometric device over a wide range of arm circumferences. Hypertens Res 2010;33:1186–91.

33. Nielsen PE, Janniche H. The accuracy of auscultatory measurement of arm blood pressure in very obese subjects. Acta Med Scand 1974;195:403–9.

34. Palatini P, Parati G. Blood pressure measurement in very obese patients: a challenging problem. J Hypertens 2011;29:425–9.

35. Ogedegbe G, Pickering T. Principles and techniques of blood pressure measurement. Cardiol Clin 2010;28(4):571–86.

36. Pickering TG, Hall JE, Appel LJ, et al. Recommendations for blood pressure measurement in humans and experimental animals: part 1: blood pressure measurement in humans: a statement for professional and public education of the American Heart Association council on high blood pressure research. Hypertension 2005;45:142–61. Available at: http://hyper.ahajournals.org/content/45/1/142. Accessed October 9, 2013.

37. Tholl T, Forstner K, Anlauf M. Measuring blood pressure: pitfalls and recommendations. Nephrol Dial Transplant 2004;19:766–70.

38. Netea RT, Lenders JW, Smits P. Both body and arm position significantly influence blood pressure measurement. J Hum Hypertens 2003;17:459.

39. Baun J. Physical principles of general and vascular sonography. San Francisco (CA): ProSono; 2014.

40. Tachovsky B. Indirect auscultatory blood pressure measurement at two sites in the arm. Res Nurs Health 1985;8(2):125–9.

41. Singer AJ, Kahn SR, Thode HC, et al. Comparison of forearm and upper arm blood pressure. Prehosp Emerg Care 1999;3:123–6.

42. Pierin AM, Alavarce DC, Gusmao JL, et al. Blood pressure measurement in obese patients: comparison between upper arm and forearm measurements. Blood Press Monit 2004;9(3):101–5.

43. Schell KA, Richards JG, Farquhar WB. The effects of anatomical structures on adult forearm and upper arm noninvasive blood pressures. Blood Press Monit 2007;12(1):17–22.

44. Schell KA, Waterhouse JK. Comparison of forearm and upper arm: automatic, noninvasive blood pressures in college students. Internet J Adv Nurs Prac 2007;9(1). http://dx.doi.org/10.5580/24d6.

45. Vinyoles E, Pujol E, de la Figuer M, et al. Measuring blood pressure in the forearm of obese patients: concordance with arm measurement. Med Clin (Barc) 2005;124(6):213–4.

46. Schell K, Lyons D, Bradley E, et al. Clinical comparison of automatic, noninvasive measurements of blood pressure in the forearm and upper arm with the patient supine or with the head of the bed raised 45: a follow-up study. Am J Crit Care 2006;15:196–205.

47. Schell K, Morse K, Waterhouse JK. Forearm and upper-arm oscillometric blood pressure comparison in acutely ill adults. West J Nurs Res 2010;32:322–40.

48. Domiano KL, Hinck SM, Savinske DL, et al. Comparison of upper arm and forearm blood pressure. Clin Nurs Res 2008;17:241–50.

49. Leblanc ME, Croteau S, Ferland A, et al. Blood pressure assessment in severe obesity: validation of a forearm approach. Obesity (Silver Spring) 2013;21: E533–41.

50. Milmaniene M, Cormillot A, Sarcona E, et al. Forearm blood pressure measurement: comparison with arm measurement. J Hypertens 2005;23:S37–8.

51. Arcuri EA, Rosa SC, Scanavini R, et al. Arm and forearm blood pressure measurements as a function of cuff width. Acta Paul Enferm 2009;22(1):37–42.

52. Trout KW, Bertrand CA, Williams MH. Measurement of blood pressure in obese persons. JAMA 1956;162:970–1.

53. Blackburn H, Kihlberg J, Brozek J. Arm versus forearm blood pressure in obesity. Am Heart J 1965;69:423–4.

54. Schell K, Bradley E, Bucher L, et al. Clinical comparison of automatic, noninvasive measurements of blood pressure in the forearm and upper arm. Am J Crit Care 2005;14:232–41.

55. Bland JM, Altman DG. Statistical methods for assessing agreement between two methods of clinical measurement. Lancet 1986;1(8476):307–10. Available at: http://www.ncbi.nim.nih.gov/pubmed/2868172. Accessed April 3, 2013.

56. Davis J, Davis I, Bennink LD, et al. Are automatic blood pressure measurements accurate in trauma patients? J Trauma 2003;55:860–3.

57. Braam RL, Thein T. Is the accuracy of blood pressure measuring devices underestimated at increasing blood pressure levels? Blood Press Monit 2005; 10:283–9.

58. Parker SB, Steigerwalk SP. The Dinamap dilemma: inaccuracy of the commonly used Dinamap 8100 compared to simultaneous mercury manometer measurement in hospitalized patients at different levels of blood pressure. Am J Hypertens 2004;17:S52.

59. Association for the Advancement of Medical Instrumentation. American national standard non-invasive sphygmomanometers-part 2: clinical validation of automated measurement type. Arlington (VA): ANSI/AAMI/ISO 81060–2; 2009. p. 1–38.

60. Spot vital signs 420 series operator's manual. Beaverton (OR): Welch Allyn; 2001.

61. Dinamap compact monitor operation manual. Tampa (FL): Critikon; 1998.

62. Netea RT, Lenders J, Smits P, et al. Influence of body and arm position on blood pressure readings: an overview. J Hypertens 2003;21:237–41.

63. Chittester B. Medical device clinical trials – how do they compare to drug trials? MasterControl Gxp Lifeline. 2014. Available at: www.mastercontrolinc.blogspot. com Accessed July 29, 2014.

64. U.S. Food and Drug Administration. Inside clinical trials: Testing medical products in people. FDA. 2013. Available at: www.fda.gov/drugs/resourcesforyou/consumers/ucm143531.htm. Accessed July 29, 2014.

65. American Nurses Association. The nurse's role in ethics and human rights: protecting and promoting individual worth, dignity, and human rights in practice settings. 2010. Available at: www.nursingworld.org/Ethics. Accessed July 29, 2014.

66. American Association of Nurse Anesthetists. Standards of nurse anesthesia practice. Available at: www.aana.com/resources2/professionalpractice/Documents. Accessed February 14, 2014.

67. Nichols WW. Clinical measurement of arterial stiffness obtained from noninvasive pressure waveforms. Am J Hypertens 2005;18:3S–10S.

68. Fonseca-Reyes S, de Alba-Garcia JG, Parra-Carillo JZ, et al. Effect of standard cuff on blood pressure readings in patients with obese arms: how frequent are arms of a "large-circumference"? Blood Press Monit 2003;8(3):101–6.

69. Ogunnaike BO, Whitten CW. Anesthesia and obesity. In: Barash PG, Cullen BF, Stoelting RK, editors. Clinical anesthesia. Philadelphia: Lippincott Williams & Wilkins; 2006. p. 1040–52.

70. Araghi A, Bander JJ, Guzman JA. Arterial blood pressure monitoring in overweight critically ill patients: invasive or noninvasive? Crit Care 2006;10(2):R64.

71. Kriz P. Obesity and anesthesia: WHEC practice bulletin and clinical management guidelines for healthcare providers. Women's Health and Education Center (WHEC). 2013. Available at: http://www.womenshealthsection.com/content/print. php3?titile=obspm008&lng=english. Accessed March 16, 2014.

72. Umana E, Ahmed W, Fraley M. Comparison of oscillometric and intra-arterial systolic and diastolic blood pressure in lean, overweight and obese patients. Angiology 2006;57(1):41–5.

Technology and Monitoring Patients at the Bedside

Benjamin A. Smallheer, PhD, RN, ACNP-BC, CCRN[a,b,*]

KEYWORDS

- Nursing • Technology • Bedside • Health care impact • Patient care technology
- ICU • Nursing care • Medical technology

KEY POINTS

- Bedside nursing plays a significant role in the adoption of new technologies incorporated within the hospital environment.
- Organizational turbulence is a result of the failure to demonstrate usability and utility of new technologies implemented into clinical practice.
- Acceptance of technology in the health care setting depends on end-user satisfaction and perceptions of usability and usefulness of medical advances.

INTRODUCTION

Over the past 5 decades, patient care technology and monitoring within the hospital environment have experienced rapid growth and advancement (**Table 1**). Much of this explosive progression has fueled the growth of critical care medicine within the intensive care unit (ICU). With the expansion of critical care medicine, so have the job responsibilities and autonomy of the bedside nurse expanded both within and outside of the intensive care environment.

Unfortunately, in recent years, despite the continued advances and improvements to technology, health care in the United States has received much criticism for being fragmented, expensive, unsafe, and unfair.[1] It is through continued commitment to the advancements in technology that improvements in quality, communication, resource utilization, and accountability hope to be achieved[1]; with the bedside nurse at the helm of these changes.

Disclosures: None.
[a] School of Nursing, Vanderbilt University School of Nursing, 461 21st Avenue South, 305 Godchaux Hall, Nashville, TN 37240, USA; [b] Pulmonary Intensivist/Rapid Response Team, St. Thomas West Hospital, 4220 Harding Road, Nashville, TN 37205, USA
* School of Nursing, Vanderbilt University School of Nursing, 461 21st Avenue South, 305 Godchaux Hall, Nashville, TN 37240.
E-mail address: benjamin.a.smallheer@vanderbilt.edu

Table 1
Timeline of technology advances in medicine

Date	Innovative Discovery
1800s	Rudimentary peritoneal dialysis performed
1887	Advancements in cardiac monitoring
1923	First PD clinical application
1929	First right heart catheter
1929	Negative pressure ventilation as a result of the polio epidemic
1943	Dialysis to treat malignant hypertension and renal failure
1945	Dialysis as a lifesaving therapy for renal failure
1950	First echo; one dimensional axial view
1950s	First volume ventilators
1952	PPV became considered when limitations of NPV were realized: expense, size, inability to secure an airway, pulmonary atelectasis
1960s	First CVP monitor
1970s	Development of the 2D echo
1970s	Introduction of Seldinger technique for percutaneous cannulation of central vessels
1970s	Development of the transesophageal echocardiogram
1972	Development of modern photoplethysmography to isolate the pulsatile variations in oxygenated and deoxygenated hemoglobin
1977	Continual renal replacement therapy via continuous arteriovenous hemofiltration
1980	Modern day pulse ox, migrated out of OR and into the ICU in 1983
1980s	Color flow Doppler; use in cardiogenic and septic shock, tamponade, aortic dissection patient
1980s	PSV developed
1983	Pulse oximeter migrated from the OR to the ICU

Abbreviations: 2D, two-dimensional; CVP, central venous pressure; echo, echocardiogram; ICU, intensive care unit; NPV, negative pressure ventilation; OR, operating room; ox, oximetry; PD, peritoneal dialysis; PPV, positive pressure ventilation; PSV, pressure support ventilation.

Data from Hannibal GB. It started with Einthoven: the history of the ECG and cardiac monitoring. AACN Adv Crit Care 2011;22(1):93–6; and Puri N, Puri V, Dellinger RP. History of technology in the intensive care unit. Crit Care Clin 2009;25:185–200.

REASON FOR TECHNOLOGY ADVANCEMENT

Technology at the bedside has continued to develop over the years, driven by the need to have a more financially responsible utilization of resources, improved quality of care, less adverse drug events, clear delineation of operational roles, improved staff and patient satisfaction, and a reduction in hospital mortality.[2,3] Technology advancements, however, should enhance the clinician's abilities and efficiency, and not be used to replace the clinician or substitute for critical thinking.[2] Computer technology has created new and innovative ways to improve data evaluation and accessibility, manage large numbers of patients simultaneously, identify emerging clinical problems, and warn of potential errors in treatment plan.[2]

Most health care workers view technology within their field as the medications, the development of new treatment plans, the equipment for direct patient care or supportive purposes, and the medical/surgical procedures.[4] Therefore, when a change in health care technology occurs, it often creates "organizational turbulence."[4] This organizational turbulence is often the result of a resistance to change and a fear of the unknown.

The nurse is the clinician who is in closest contact with the patient for the greatest sustained period of time. Therefore, the greatest level of interaction with both the patient and the technology associated with the patients' care is also experienced by the nurse.[5] Within nurses' daily interactions, a great amount of specialized and individualized knowledge is necessary. A workable knowledge of the patients' biophysical and psychological responses to illness is required. This knowledge, which constitutes "knowing a patient," cannot be gained from technology alone.

Trust is defined as a behavior, an attitude, an intention, or a belief in the reliability, skill, or strength of someone or something.[5] Therefore, it is not uncommon that with the introduction of a new technology aimed at "make the nurse's job easier" skepticism on the part of the nurse is experienced. A lack of trust may be felt based on the distance the technology places between the clinician and the physiologic/psychological experiences of the patient. The ability to interact with these experiences is the cornerstone of nursing practice.[4]

INSTITUTION OF NEW TECHNOLOGY

The institution of new technology within the medical setting requires a certain amount of time and attention by the end-user. Who is this end-user? It is the medical personnel: nurses, nurse practitioners, physician assistants, physicians, and all other members of the medical team who might interact with the technology.

In order for the clinician to fully adopt the change in technology, there must be a perception of (1) usability of the technology and (2) utility or usefulness of the technology.[6] Usability and usefulness are therefore key elements of end-user satisfaction. End-user satisfaction is defined as "the affective attitude towards a specific computer application by someone who interacts with the application directly"[7] and is a critical factor of information technology implementation. This satisfaction is highly dependent on the technologies' usability, usefulness, and efficiency within a specified context of use. Finally, the end-user must have trust in the technology. Without trust in the ability of the technology to fulfill its goal, clinicians are less likely to embrace and welcome the change.

The tasks of "maintenance and upkeep" for technology, however, can be seen as difficult, laborious, and demanding. The more time a nurse spends tending to the machines, the less time is spent nurturing the holistic needs of the patient.[4] Historically, nurses in the 1970s were troubled by the intrusion of technology into their field. Nurses, who dedicated their lives to serving the ill, injured, and unfortunate, began to view the introduction of technology as an obstacle to providing patient care.[4] Their hands were being taken off the patient and placed onto devices that were being introduced as a way to make their jobs easier and more efficient.

In today's health care society, because of nursing shortages and increased demands in the work environment, novice nurses are often forced to learn superficial survival skills that enslave them to technology rather than to learn how to master technology and patient care.[4] Becoming too depending on the technology, however, poses a significant risk. If the equipment fails to carry out its function or does not alert human operators of changes in system status, catastrophic outcomes may ensue. Such adverse consequences are not specific to nursing and have been seen in other disciplines, which incorporate heavy dependence on technology: aviation, shipping, and nuclear and chemical industries.[5] Operators of the technology develop blind trust and often dependence on a piece of equipment. This trust and dependence can cause an overestimation in the technologies' reliability and, as a consequence, second check systems or independent assessments are not used.[5]

TECHNOLOGIES OF THE NEW MILLENNIUM

Since the new millennium, numerous technologies have arisen at the bedside, benefiting nurses and physicians alike. These technologies, although intended to streamline nursing responsibilities, patient care, and documentation, have been received with varying levels of acceptance.

Point of Care

The movement to bring technology and monitoring to the client's bedside can most readily be seen through the use of handheld point-of-care (POC) testing devices.[8] Over the past 20 years, POC, defined as medical testing at or near the site of the patient, has intended to bring the laboratory testing to the patient in both a convenient and a rapid manner.[9] By doing so, patient compliance, obtaining of test results, as well as a more expeditious plan of care can be made.

Early medicine was conducted at the bedside, usually in the patient's home. With the improvement of technologies and modalities of care, patients were eventually brought to hospitals and the use of centralized laboratories became recognized as conventional practice. This transition away from home care and into institutionalized care saw a decrease in the use of POC testing. The re-emergence of POC testing continues to grow as the need for critical treatment plans are dependent on laboratory results. In today's bedside practice, nurses are using POC testing regularly to guide patient care in areas such as blood glucose management, acid-base interpretation, and progression of care following procedures such as angioplasty (**Box 1**).[10]

These devices have been readily adopted and embraced by bedside nurses. Through the use of POC testing, the typical process of sending a blood specimen to the laboratory and waiting up to an hour for results to determine the next step in the treatment plan has been altered. By decreasing this wait time to minutes, (1) minimal delay in care is experienced and (2) patients experience decreased anxiety while awaiting the results.

Automated Dispensing Systems

Automatic dispensing systems emerged in the mid 1990s in Europe as a means to help community pharmacies improve dispensing time. A large pharmacy's inventory could easily exceed 5000 items, causing time delays and inefficient staff utilization if an individual needed to retrieve each item by hand. Therefore, a robotic dispensary system was developed to make the job of the pharmacist more efficient.

Although these initial machines were not intended for use in the hospital setting, the implications for use and the impact on patient safety through minimizing adverse drug events was recognized. The technology was eventually modified and transitioned to the nursing units. These machines would store medications through a variety of ways and organizational systems until needed by the nurse.

Before the institution of medication dispensing machines on the nursing unit, either a rolling cart with a series of drawers or a cabinet in a medication room was frequently used to store the patient's ordered medications. The cart and/or the drawers may or may not have had a locking system. Narcotics were stored in a similar drawer design with a signature sheet for administration and waste. A refrigerator was used to store items that needed to be temperature controlled. These systems required the nurse to find a patient's medications within the drawer system and administer the medication with little ability to double check what was being given or the dosage.

In modern day nursing practice, the standard of care is for facilities to have medications housed in a medication dispensing system where staff can gain access through

Box 1
Laboratory tests available through point of care technology

Aspartate aminotransferase

Bladder tumor-associated antigen

Blood glucose testing

Brain natriuretic peptide

Cholesterol screening

C-reactive protein

Drugs of abuse screening

Electrolytes analysis

Fecal occult blood analysis

Follicle-stimulating hormone

Food pathogens screening

Helicobacter pylori

Hemoglobin A1c

Hemoglobin/hematocrit

HIV salivary assay

Homocysteine

Human chorionic gonadotropin/pregnancy testing

Infectious disease testing

Influenza A and B

Ketones

Lipoprotein testing

Lithium drug levels

Liver function

Luteinizing hormone and Fern test

Microalbumin

Mononucleosis

Prothrombin time/international normalized ratio

Rapid cardiac markers diagnostics

Renal function

Reproductive testing

Respiratory syncytial virus

Streptococcus

Trichomonas

Triglycerides

Urine dipstick testing

Vaginal pH and amines

Data from Refs.[8–10]

the use of user-specific login and password. Medications are then profiled for each patient after an appropriate order is reviewed and confirmed by a Doctor of Pharmacy. A small number of medications deemed to have indications in an emergency situation are available in an "override" capacity, although the safety checks used by the machine are not engaged with this function.[2,11]

For the bedside nurse, the current process of accessing medications through a dispensing system is slower; however, the safety checks used have exponential benefits. Not only is there added protection for the patient against potential adverse drug events and other medication errors but also the nurse has a layer of protection as well against potential medication errors and litigation. Along with the safety aspects of dispensing medication systems, barcode scanning technology also contributes to medication administration safety and a decrease in adverse drug events. This technology will be discussed later.

Electronic Medication Records

Utilization of electronic medication records (EMR) has become the standard of practice. What used to be either handwritten or computer printed daily is being replaced by a real-time, computerized version that synchronizes to the active orders within the patient's chart. Both of these older methods required manual signatures, initials, handwritten, or highlighted entries for medication additions or discontinuations mid shift.

In many facilities, large numbers of medication errors are what prompted an increased interest in using technology to improve medication administration safety. With the proper institution of technology, a reduction in adverse drug events shows great potential.[2] The complexity of an EMR, however, is even more pronounced in an ICU setting because of the rapidly changing medication needs and unique dosing requirements of the patient population.[2] These requirements often demand the presence of a critical care pharmacist to help guide and dose the medical therapies being requested by the Intensivist team.

Currently, the usage of EMR by bedside nurses has streamlined the process of medication administration and reconciliation. The bedside nurse is typically responsible for entering home medications into the patient's electronic health record (EHR). The provider, then, has the ability to continue those medications while in the hospital, sometimes with one simple keystroke. Likewise, the provider can opt to not continue a medication. During the discharge process, the provider is able to generate discharge medication reconciliation from the active inpatient EMR with a similar keystroke. This procedure has greatly decreased the workload of the nurse in the handwritten construction of such reconciliations along with the potential for errors in transcription or legibility. Finally, having the oversight of a pharmacist within the hospital setting during this process dramatically impacts patient safety.

Electronic Health Record

Following the implementation of the EMR was the transition to a full EHR. Although sounding a bit minimized, the task of creating a fully EHR is quite expansive and requires an interdisciplinary approach and design. Implementation and use of EHR technology have raised numerous challenges, including end-user acceptance.[6] With the institution of this technology, if nurses found the EHR technology neither usable nor useful, negative perceptions and attitudes toward the technology would develop, and continued use of the system's full features and adoption would pose a significant challenge.

A large benefit to the institution of the EHR is readily seen on the data management side of the facility. No longer are large rooms needed for storing medical records in paper form. Medical records can now be stored electronically, and any existing paper charts are able to be scanned into the new EHR for their respective patients. When old records are needed at the bedside for review by the clinicians, requests to medical records departments are no longer needed, and files no longer need to be delivered from what was often an offsite location. Rather, the current plan of care can be reinforced through a simple search within the patient's EHR. The time delays once experienced have been minimized to seconds. This benefit has also been observed when a patient is transferred between hospitals within a particular health system. Staff is able to directly view the records electronically from those facilities, eliminating the need for sending facilities to print records and copy radiographic studies to DVD for transfer: all having the potential of getting lost or damaged.

Additional benefits can be seen in transcription and readability of documents. Providers are often rushed and use a form of shorthand when manually documenting in a paper record. Illegible handwriting has been shown to be 1 of the 5 top contributors to medication errors.[12] Using computer technology can aid in readability of all records, and improved comprehension of the plan of care.

These benefits to the EHR, however, are not always embraced by the bedside staff. Previously, with the handwritten health record, the bedside nurse could freely handwrite a nursing note, describing the nursing assessment and findings. This manner of free writing allowed for the expression of thought and ideas using a SOAP (Subjective, Objective, Assessment, Plan) format. Using the EHR, nurses often find themselves searching through the assessment database and its multiple dropdown menus, looking for the precise way to describe the findings, or the interventions that were conducted.

A phenomenon known to nurses as "double charting" has also arisen. Standard nursing practice is for the bedside clinician to only have to document a particular finding at one location within the health record. With the institution of EHR, particular findings are required to be charted in numerous locations due to overlap in body systems and treatment modalities. The practice of double charting can pose great frustration to the nursing staff and divert time away from patient care and into navigating the charting system.

Radiography Technology

Traditionally, radiograph technology required the nurse to transport the patient to the radiology department to obtain the ordered radiography study. The process of having the film developed, interpreted by a qualified provider, and then having the results communicated to either the ordering provider or ultimately the nurse produced significant delays in care. Although the first portable radiography machines date back to World War I, the advanced benefits were noted following the introduction of radiograph digitalization in the United States in 1983.[13]

With advances in the methods of obtaining radiographs, portable radiography machines became digitized and allowed providers to view images seconds after being obtained. In addition, with the use of PACS (picture archiving and communication systems), providers are able to view the image outside of the radiology department. Providers may be in an office, on a patient care unit, or even at home, and still able to log into the system to review the radiograph.

Furthermore, the portable nature of viewing these images has allowed nurses and providers alike to take these test results to the bedside. In the ICU, this translates to more efficient endotracheal tube placement confirmation, ruling out of pneumothorax, and central line placement. Outside the ICU, concerns for pneumonia, feeding tube placement, and imaging of injuries and aliments can be expedited. This ability to bring both the medical testing and the results to the patient has the potential to improve comprehension, compliance, and the development of a more client-centered plan of care.

Previously, a provider may have attempted to describe or draw an image or diagnostic finding. Now, images can be shown to the patient and family for improved understanding. In addition, nurses are able to help facilitate care and assure all the patient's questions and concerns are addressed.

Computerized Provider Order Entry

One of the final steps in converting health records to an electronic format is computerized provider/physician order entry (CPOE). The Leapfrog Group in 2008 presented several key recommendations to support safety, quality, and affordability of health care. One specific recommendation included the application of CPOE systems.[3] The primary goals of CPOE as stated by the Leapfrog Group are as follows:

- Prompting or warning providers against the possibility of drug interaction, allergy, or overdose
- Supplying current information that helps providers keep up with new drugs entering the market
- Supplying drug-specific information that eliminates confusion among drug names that sound alike
- Improving communication between providers and pharmacists
- Reducing health care costs due to improved efficiency[14]

As of 2010 though, only 15% of US hospitals had implemented CPOE. CPOE experienced previous failures due to a lack of usability, usefulness, and the development of safety problems with its application.[7]

CPOE requires ordering providers to specify many aspects of orders that may have previously been completed by nurses, pharmacists, and others. This new system places a greater responsibility and accountability on the ordering individual, relieving the nurses from the burden of interpreting and contacting providers to clarify orders.[7] Likewise, the intent of CPOE is to minimize the involvement of third-party individuals, such as the nursing staff, when orders are being entered.

Providers tended to be more satisfied with the CPOE system than bedside nurses. Along with the dramatic benefits of the CPOE system, numerous unanticipated difficulties have been encountered. Providers can enter orders from other locations within the hospital and elsewhere, making verbal orders less necessary.[6] Nurses experienced difficulty with the provider's ability to enter orders from remote locations because of:

- An unawareness of new orders being entered
- Less face-to-face communication between nurse and provider
- A possibility of provider to patient interaction being lost

Another concern experienced by bedside nurses surrounds the time delay of receiving admission orders. Many providers would previously give orders over the telephone and/or verbally to allow care for the patient to begin. In the current culture surrounding CPOE, telephone/verbal orders are minimized. What was intended to be a streamlined process now leaves nurses waiting for the admitting provider to enter orders for the patient. This time delay may be minimal but may also span several hours, forcing the nurse to improvise before a firm plan of care is decided on and ordered.

Computer on Wheels/Workstation on Wheels

Through the progression of technology and its direct impact on bedside nursing, the need to bring care and technology to the bedside has continued to surge. This surge has facilitated the development and increased utilization of Computer on Wheels/ Workstation on Wheels (COW/WOW) within direct patient care areas. This achievement would have been hindered if not for technology advancements in computer portability. The computers of the 1990s or even 2000s would have been less suited for the needed mobility when compared with the currently available hardware and battery life.

In current times, COWs/WOWs have allowed providers to bring patient care into the room where originally it was limited by landline power cords to the nurses' station or dictation rooms. Physician and Intensivist rounds can now be conducted at the bedside with the patient's radiographs, EMR, and EHR present, which originally was not possible. This change in culture has allowed the patient and family to both become part of the decision-making process surrounding the plan of care. Patients and families can see laboratory results, hear discussions within a multidisciplinary team, review radiographs with the providers, and engage in holistic health decisions.

COWs/WOWs have a huge impact on bedside nursing care. Previously, the nurses dedicated much time to detective work: chasing down providers, digging through the medical chart, deciphering poor penmanship, and helping the patient understand what all the members of the health care team were thinking. Now, all individuals can come together into a single conversation and assure adequate and holistic patient care is provided with all questions answered.

Once the mobility of access had been addressed, further use of barcode scanning for medication administration became available.[2,6] The culmination of the EMR and EHR allowed an integrative system, whereby the bedside nurse is able to scan the barcode on each unit dose of medication to be administered as well as scanning a barcode on the patient's identification band. Both of these scanned items then correlate with the patient's EMR to confirm the correct patient, correct medication, correct dose, correct route, and correct time. The confirmed 5 rights of medication administration greatly decrease the potential for adverse drug events.

Smart Pump Technology

Devices often overlooked as having technology advancement are the infusion pumps and hemodynamic monitoring equipment. Even as recent as 10 years ago, these devices used a much more simplistic internal program and were unable to perform many of the tasks for which they are depended on in modern patient care. Traditional infusion pumps required the bedside nurse to enter a program based on milliliters per hour and a volume to be infused, also in milliliters per hour. These programs were vulnerable to errors in not only the administration of the medications being given but also the monitoring of the medication.[2,6,15] In addition, charting of infusions required sometimes intricate calculations by the nurse to account for rate changes, temporary interruptions in infusions, or discontinuations at an inconvenient time.

Smart pump technology exists in most new model infusion pumps. These devices are programmed with numerous soft stops, which prompt the user to reconsider an entered dose, or hard stops, which prevent the user from going beyond a particular programmed limit.[15] By doing so, adverse drug events are minimized and a series of checks and balances are provided. Many pumps also contain embedded software programs that help guide the bedside nurse into proper infusion of medications. This software may be specifically set based on patient weight, unit protocols within a facility (limiting chemotherapy medications outside of oncology units), or the extent of care being provided to a patient (general care unit vs ICU). These programs help minimize overdosing or infusions at inappropriate rates.

Like the smart pumps, many noninvasive hemodynamic monitoring devices have been developed with technology to populate the patient's EHR. By scanning a patient's identification band barcode, these machines are able to automatically upload temperature, blood pressure, heart rate, and pulse oximetry to the patient's chart.

Both of these devices have greatly improved the work of the bedside nurse, but not without the occasional complication. Automatic charting of infusions and vital signs is a time-saving action for the nurse though; the potential for erroneous information to be uploaded to the EHR is possible. Often, the nurse must review and verify each value to assure accuracy. In addition, concerning vital signs may be missed as a result of unlicensed health care personnel not having the educational background to understand the severity of a reading and uploading the values without alerting the bedside nurse.

Telemedicine

Instituted more than 25 years ago, telemedicine has developed an intricate and elaborate commercial application.[2,16] An additional key recommendation by the Leapfrog Group was to include an increase in ICU physician staffing.[3] With the limited availability of Intensivist trained providers, telemedicine made available an option for medical facilities with limited access to specialty trained teams. Telemedicine is an on-demand means of networking critical care consultants with facilities lacking Intensivist specialists.[3] This concept was initially designed to provide care through remote monitoring. The ability to intervene, however, was generally instituted when necessary, causing care to be provided in a reactive manner rather than a proactive one.[16]

Telemedicine has been associated with lower mortality both within ICUs over time and across ICUs during the same period.[16] The use of telemedicine has also been extending beyond the ICU and into the Emergency Department, Rapid Response Teams, High-Risk Labor and Delivery Units, and Long-Term Acute Care Hospitals.[3]

Telemedicine has been shown to be a beneficial technology on both the side of the provider and the bedside nursing frontier. More clear direction can be given to the bedside nurse regarding a treatment plan, allowing for a more thorough implementation of the plan of care. In addition, by having access to expert clinicians, nurses can model their practice after the efficient practice of an Intensivist service.

THE NURSE'S PERSPECTIVE

When candidly asking seasoned nurses about the impact of technology on the role of the bedside nurse, a variety of thoughts surfaced. Several shared the benefits of technology, whereas others insinuated a loss of independent thought by the nurse.

Positive Impact

- Legal protection is improved due to computerized charting
- Improved ventilator modes and advanced therapies
- Provider can view charts from other locations
- Improved security through login and server advancements
- EMR/barcode scanning is safer and improved
- Ease in obtaining and viewing intrafacility records

Negative Impact

- Takes longer to chart
- More to chart
- Numerous dropdown boxes
- Software frequently cannot keep up with hardware

- More time is spent on the computer
- Developed by nonclinicians
- Takes away from patient care: bath versus charting

TECHNOLOGY YET TO COME

With all the technology that has been achieved, it would seem there is little more to be accomplished. Therefore, what is on the forefront of technology to improve bedside nursing? The application of genetics/genomics in health care continues to be researched. Within a health care society centered on genetics, providers can more efficiently use therapies consistent with the metabolism and receptors of the patient being treated. This tailored medical practice can be achieved without the typical trial and error method currently used. More accurate and specialized health care translates to more efficient care provided by the bedside nurse.

Mobile technology will take a greater role in health care. Current developments of health promotion applications for mobile devices have the ability to synchronize to larger programs, keeping track of physical activity, dietary intake, and sleep patterns. Handheld mobile devices will no longer be only for communication and social media but a gateway to individual health care.

Therapies will become faster, more efficient, and less invasive. These advances will drastically minimize hospital length of stay and capitalize on home recovery, where the environment is predictable and stable. With all these potential advancements, however, the rising cost of health care will no longer be able to be ignored. Improved technology is accompanied by a more expensive bottom line.

SUMMARY

Advances in technology have brought the bedside nurse a great distance from the days of Florence Nightingale. Her insight was revolutionary and brilliant given her lack of technology. In comparison to today's health care model, the quality goal to be achieved will be unattainable if not engaged within a team effort. "A coordinated multidisciplinary team working with healthcare technology will elevate us to our desired outcomes".[2] Sitting at the front line providing holistic care, while holding the hand of the patient, is the bedside nurse. If new technologies do not make the nurses' job more efficient, the compassionate care nurses strive to deliver will be consumed by tasks, check boxes, and key strokes.

REFERENCES

1. Amarasingham R, Plantinga L, Diener-West M, et al. Clinical information technologies and inpatient outcomes. Arch Intern Med 2009;169(2):108–14.
2. Hassan E, Badawi O, Weber RJ, et al. Using technology to prevent adverse drug events in the intensive care unit. Crit Care Med 2010;38(6):S97–105.
3. Jarrah S, Van der Kloot TE. Tele-ICU: remote critical care telemedicine. American College of Chest Physicians web site. 2010. Available at: http://69.36.35.38/accp/pccsu/tele-icu-remote-critical-care-telemedicine?page=0,3. Accessed September 1, 2014.
4. Crocker C, Timmons S. The role of technology in critical care nursing. J Adv Nurs 2009;65(1):52–61.
5. Browne M, Cook P. Inappropriate trust in technology: implications for critical care nurses. Nurs Crit Care 2011;16(2):92–8.

6. Carayon P, Cartmill R, Blosky MA, et al. ICU nurses' acceptance of electronic health records. J Am Med Inform Assoc 2011;18:812–9.

7. Hoonakker PL, Carayon P, Walker JM. Measurement of COPE end-user satisfaction among ICU physicians and nurses. Appl Clin Inform 2010;1(3):268–85.

8. Facts sheet: point-of-care diagnostic. National Institute of Health web site. 2010. Available at: http://report.nih.gov/nihfactsheets/Pdfs/PointofCareDiagnostic Testing(NIBIB).pdf. Accessed October 13, 2014.

9. Nichols JH. Point of care testing. Clin Lab Med 2007;27:893–908.

10. Point of care testing toolkit. College of American Pathologists web site. 2013. Available at: http://www.cap.org/apps/cap.portal?_nfpb=true&cntvwrPtlt_action Override=%2Fportlets%2FcontentViewer%2Fshow&_windowLabel=cntvwrPtlt& cntvwrPtlt%7BactionForm.contentReference%7D=committees%2Fpointofcare %2Fpoc_toolkit_history.html&_state=maximized&_pageLabel=cntvwr. Accessed November 10, 2014.

11. Facts about automated dispensing. Willach Pharmacy Solutions Web site. 2010. Available at: http://willach-pharmacy-solutions.com/au/news/press/Facts-about-automated-dispensing.phpPublished. Accessed October 24, 2014.

12. Jones JH, Treiber L. When the 5 rights go wrong: medication errors from the nursing perspective. J Nurs Care Qual 2010;25(3):240–7.

13. Frederick Jones Biography. Available at: http://www.biography.com/people/frederick-jones-21329957. Accessed November 5, 2014.

14. Facts sheet: computerized physician order entry. The Leapfrog Group. 2014. Available at: http://www.leapfroghospitalsurvey.org. Accessed September 25, 2014.

15. Reston J. Smart pumps and other protocols for infusion pumps: brief review. In: Making health care safer II: an updated critical analysis of the evidence for patient safety practices. Santa Monica (CA): RAND; 2013. p. 48–54.

16. Kahn JM. The use and misuse of ICU telemedicine. JAMA 2011;305(21):2227–8.

Transforming Home Health Nursing with Telehealth Technology

Francisca Cisneros Farrar, EdD, MSN, RN

KEYWORDS

- Home health nursing • Mental health nurse role • Telehealth technology
- Recovery model • Evidence-based tool • Ethical considerations
- Legal considerations • Electronic personal health records

KEY POINTS

- The historical transition of mental health care from a rehabilitation model to recovery model has transformed the home health nursing role in providing care for mental health patients.
- Cognitive behavior therapy restructures patients' thinking with positive reinforcement and natural consequences to develop adaptive behavior and is the conceptual framework and technological framework for Telehealth interventions.
- Research validates Telehealth technology as an evidence-based delivery tool for mental health.
- Telehealth technology supplementing a mental health skilled nurse visit can facilitate shared decision making, empower collaborative care, and help maintain patients in the home setting.
- Ethical guidelines need to be followed when supplementing mental health care with Telehealth technology.
- Federal and state laws govern Telehealth technology and nurses must be abreast of current laws/policies that could impact their practice.

INTRODUCTION

The shift from institutional treatment to the community care setting for mental health patients has increased the demand for home health services to maintain patients in the community.[1] The historical transition of mental health care from a rehabilitation

Disclosures: None.
Conflict of Interest: None.
School of Nursing, Austin Peay State University, ffig601 College Street, Clarksville, TN 37044, USA
E-mail address: farrarf@apsu.edu

model to the recovery model has transformed the home health nursing role in providing care for mental health patients. The recovery model promotes family support and partnership in a collaborative approach to treatment of mental illness to maintain patients in the community.[2] Studies show the use of telemonitoring devices, such as remotely monitoring physiologic and psychological variables, are effective in reducing the need for readmission and are useful tools for trending data for decision making.[3] Mental health nurses need to be aware of emerging technology to provide cutting-edge evidence-based care to keep mental health patients in the community setting. This article provides an update on Telehealth technology used in the mental health setting. This article presents the historical transformation of delivery models for the home setting, discusses how cognitive behavioral therapy is used as the conceptual and behavioral framework for Telehealth behavior interventions, presents research examples to validate Telehealth is an evidence-based delivery tool, and points out ethical considerations in using Telehealth technology. The article provides an overview of legal considerations with using these tools, describes how Telehealth has transformed the mental health nurse role, provides examples of applications of Telehealth to integrate into a plan of care for mental health patients and management of coexisting medical chronic comorbidities, describes how health literacy can impact patients' understanding of their electronic personal health records, and justifies why nurses need to respond to their role change by developing skill competencies for emerging technology to provide safe, quality, and accountable nursing practice to meet positive patient outcomes.

HISTORICAL TRANSFORMATION OF DELIVERY MODELS FOR THE HOME SETTING
Rehabilitation Model

Patients are admitted to the psychiatric inpatient setting based on the severity of their illness and level of dysfunction, such as patients with suicidal or homicidal ideation/actions. Some patients have involuntary inpatient admissions by the criminal justice system as a result of criminal charges for court-ordered observation and treatment of their mental illness.[1] The rehabilitation model has a focus on deficits, symptoms, and stability.[2] Patients are discharged to the community when the behavior has improved with medication and therapy. Home care services for skilled mental health nurse visits are ordered to deliver care to patients and their families to help with transition from the inpatient setting to the home setting.[3] The focus of the plan of care is rehabilitation.

Recovery Model

The consumer movement focusing on choices, empowerment, and quality of life generated the transition of mental health care from a rehabilitation model to a recovery model for the community setting. The consumer movement was influenced by the Healthy People 2020 goals and the Institute of Medicine call for collaborative care. The Healthy People 2020 goals recommend that health communication and information technology can improve population health outcomes, health care quality, and support shared decision making between patients and providers.[4] The 2010 Institute of Medicine report, *The Future of Nursing*, suggests that nurses need to master technological tools and information systems while collaborating care across interdisciplinary teams.[4] The focus of the plan of care is recovery with emphasis on empowerment with shared decision making and collaborative care. This model uses Telehealth tools to supplement the skilled mental health visits to provide collaborative care and make an informed decision.

CONCEPTUAL AND BEHAVIORAL FRAMEWORK FOR TELEHEALTH BEHAVIOR INTERVENTIONS

The recovery model uses cognitive behavioral therapy to restructure patients' thinking with positive reinforcement and natural consequences to develop adaptive behavior. Social skills training and supportive counseling also are components of this model.[2] The behavioral intervention technologies was designed as a conceptual and technological framework for Telehealth interventions, such as mobile phones, the Web, and sensors to support patients using programs for changing behaviors and cognitions related to health, mental health, and wellness.[5] This model is based on the translation of a treatment model and interventions. For example, if a goal for patients is weight loss, a fitness application (app) such as MyFitnessPal can be used. This mobile app uses monitoring of behavior change and weight loss. It allows patients to track what they eat and how much they exercise and uses behavior change strategies such as education, feedback, motivation, and goal setting.[5] This conceptual and technological framework provides evidence-based best practices for mobile apps. The use of this model demonstrates how technology can improve disease management and coping skills with their disease process.[2]

Mobile phone apps have been developed for cognitive behavioral therapy. This can supplement home health nurse visits. For example, the Touchscreen Mood Map allows patients to plot their mood and identify what circumstances cause a change in their mood. Patients or their caregiver can select therapeutic choices involving cognitive restructuring and relaxation.[2] Another example is the Mind Scan exercise involving cognitive reappraisal of thoughts, such as what led to their anger of depression.[2]

THE NATIONAL ALLIANCE OF MENTAL ILLNESS

The National Alliance of Mental Illness (NAMI) supports the recovery model for treatment in the community setting. In goal 6.1, the NAMI New Freedom Commission proposal to transform mental health care in America recommends the use of health technology and Telehealth to improve access and coordination of mental health care.[6] This Commission believes that Telehealth is a greatly underused resource for mental health services, and can increase access to care for patients with multiple chronic health conditions, severe illness, disability, and underserved populations.[6]

TYPES OF TELEHEALTH

There are 2 methods for conducting Telehealth: (1) real time and (2) store and forward. Real-time Telehealth allows participants to send and receive information instantly with little delay, such as with videoconferencing. Decisions can be made immediately and assist with a clinical consultation.[7] For example, through an interactive video, patients can call a home health nurse to ask about their depression symptoms, medications, giving their insulin injection, or their shortness of breath. Patient data are triaged and the patient can receive immediate information.[8] In store and forward, the information is encapsulated and then transmitted to the recipient for a reply, such as with Tele-radiology in which a digital X-ray image is sent by an e-mail to a radiologist for evaluation. The recipient reviews the information at his or her convenience, thereby causing a delay in a response.[7] Patient blood glucose levels and vital signs can be stored in remote monitoring devices that store and forward data to nurses who then assist patients with preventive measures to decrease complications and reduce emergency room visits.[8]

EVIDENCE-BASED DELIVERY TOOL

Evidence-based research validates that Telehealth is an evidence-based delivery tool for mental health. Research supports the use of Telehealth technology by mental health nurses to provide quality, safe, accountable, shared decision making, and collaborative care. Telehealth supplementing mental health nurses in the home setting can be a tool to increase the quality of patients' lives and help maintain them in the home setting. The following sections summarize examples of research supporting Telehealth as a credible tool for home health care.

Problem-Solving Therapy via Skype

A randomized control study was conducted on 121 homebound depressed patients who were 50 years and older to determine in-home Telehealth delivery of problem-solving therapy (tele-PST). The study compared problem-solving therapy via Skype video call to telephone support calls for 6 sessions. The depression scores of tele-PST in-person at the 12-week follow-up were significantly lower than those of telephone support calls. Participants had positive attitudes about Telehealth via Skype. The researchers concluded that Telehealth was an effective treatment modality for depressed homebound adults and would facilitate their access to treatment.[9]

Personal Digital Assistants for Bipolar Treatment

In a study of bipolar patients, the Improving Adherence in Bipolar Disorders (IABD) program was used in a mobile application. Bipolar patients were given a personal digital assistant (PDA) loaded with the IABD program. The program's goals were to encourage appointment attendance and medication compliance. The mobile application targeted knowledge, behaviors, attitudes, and beliefs. Patients received alerts to log in and complete a brief assessment about their mood, psychiatric symptoms, and medication compliance twice a day. The program analyzed data and provided messages to encourage continual treatment adherence. Results found increased compliance with the treatment program and decreased severity of depression symptoms.[10]

Remote Monitoring of Chronic Illness

Case studies of 4 community health services in England that use Telehealth to monitor patients with chronic obstructive pulmonary disease and chronic heart failure were conducted to determine frontline nurses' acceptance of Telehealth and identify barriers that exist. Thematic analysis of qualitative interviews with 84 stakeholders included nurses, managers, and other frontline staff. Staff attitudes ranged from resistance to enthusiasm. Reliable and flexible technology, clinical training, encouragement to use Telehealth, and dedicated resources were identified as measures to overcome barriers for acceptance of Telehealth. Adoption of Telehealth into routine practice was recommended.[11]

Management of Case Loads

A qualitative study was conducted to explore the use of Telehealth technology to assist case managers for managing their caseloads for patients with a diagnosis of human immunodeficiency virus/AIDS and living in a rural area.[12] Telehealth monitors were placed in 6 patients' homes for 6 months. Equipment included a provider station and a patient station. Peripheral equipment included blood pressure equipment, scale, glucometer, camera, and floor lamp.[12] At the time of the scheduled home health nurse visit, a video conference was done. The nurse was able to collect data about the patient's blood pressure, temperature, heart rate, lung sounds, blood glucose level, abdominal sounds, and weight. The nurse was also able to assess the patient's skin condition, and opportunistic infections. The patient used a diagram to help assist in placement of the peripheral equipment.[12] During the video conference call, the nurse was able to collect additional data about current medications, general health and mental status, emergency room or hospital visits, and any problems the patient may be experiencing.[12] After 4 months of Telehealth visits, the 6 patients were interviewed about their experience. They were asked about their satisfaction and the patient's perception about the use of Telehealth as a method to manage caseloads. Three themes emerged from the data analysis: (1) participants missed the physical presence of the nurse; (2) they were satisfied with the Telehealth case management visit, including mastering the equipment, being able to see the nurse in the videoconference; (3) it was an improvement over a regular telephone call, and it got the job done.[12] There were minimal drawbacks in using the equipment. The study concluded that Telehealth technology is an effective tool for effectively managing caseloads and responsiveness to patients' changing medical conditions.[12]

Telephones Are a Valuable Technological Tool

A research study was conducted to determine the effectiveness of integrating depression management into routine skilled visits of Medicare home health patients diagnosed with depression. Depression severity was assessed using the Hamilton Scale for Depression for 306 participants.[13] Home health nursing teams at 6 nationwide home health care agencies were randomly assigned to participants who would also receive the intervention of the Depression CAREPATH and participants who would not receive the intervention.[13] Nurse teams assigned to the depression intervention were trained to manage depression during routine home visits by conducting symptom assessment, medication management, care coordination, education, and goal setting.[13] Follow-up of patients was conducted at 3 months, 6 months, and 12 months for depression symptoms by research staff blinded to who was in the intervention group. Participants were interviewed at home and by telephone. Depression severity did not differ at 3 months or 6 months in the Depression CAREPATH and control groups.[13] The 12-month measurement did demonstrate effectiveness in the Depression CAREPATH group. The researchers concluded that home health nurses can effectively integrate depression into routine practice and can clinically benefit patients with moderate to severe depression. Telephone technology is a valid tool for treatment and data collection.[13]

Videoconferencing for Substance Abuse Counseling

A randomized study comparing video counseling versus in-person counseling was conducted over a 12-week period. Eighty-five patients attending an outpatient treatment program for opioid addiction were randomly put into a group in which counseling was in-person or a group in which video counseling was done.[14] Both groups received opioid maintenance therapy, drug screening, and weekly counseling sessions. A questionnaire about treatment satisfaction and therapeutic alliance rating was performed at baseline and monthly.[14] Results of the study showed no differences in the percentage of positive drug screens or compliance to attending the counseling sessions.[14] The study concluded that the use of videoconference is a feasible alternative to in-person counseling for patients with opioid dependence.[14]

ETHICAL CONSIDERATIONS

Ethical guidelines need to be followed when supplementing mental health care with Telehealth technology. The issues of technical skills, health literacy with users, and diagnosis need to be considered.[15] Patients with severe mental illness, such as schizophrenia, have cognitive changes that promote challenges in interacting with technology and in performing functional skills of daily living. Aging individuals may also have cognitive impairment and challenges with developing technological skills.[16] Telehealth technology is not an appropriate delivery tool for all patients and should be considered when supplementing home health visits with Telehealth technology. For example, patients with schizophrenia could interpret Telehealth devices as controlling their brain and exacerbate their symptoms. Older adults may lack required psychomotor skills, such as having arthritis, and/or lack cognitive skills, such as having impaired memory, to participate in home Telehealth. Patients have a right to refuse Telehealth technology being used in their plan of care. However, the home health nurse can use technological devices to access an electronic template for documentation, patient records, and communicate with the primary provider for collaborative care.

International Code of Ethics for Telehealth Technology

In 2000, the eHealth Ethics Initiative introduced an International Code of Ethics for health care sites and services on the Internet.[17] These principles apply to any organization or individual that provides health care information, products, or services online and are as follows:

- Candor: Disclose information that would impact a consumer's understanding or use of the site or purchase or use of a product or service. The services should be credible and trustworthy with no conflict of interest.[17]
- Honesty: Be truthful and not deceptive. Services and products should be described truthfully and information patients receive should not be presented in a misleading way.[17]
- Quality: Provide health information that is accurate, easy to understand, and up to date. Users have the right to accurate and well-supported information to make their own judgments about the health care information provided by the site.[17]
- Informed Consent: Respect users' right to determine whether or how their personal data may be collected, used, or shared. Users have the right to choose if they will allow their personal data to be collected and how it will be used or shared.[17]
- Privacy: Respect the obligation to protect users' privacy. Users have the right to expect that personal data they provide will be kept confidential and to know how the site stores users' personal data and for how long it stores that data.[17]
- Professionalism in Online Health Care: Respect fundamental ethical obligations to patients and clients. Abide by the ethical codes that govern their professions as practitioners in face-to-face relationships.[17]
- Responsible Partnering: Ensure that organizations and sites with which they affiliate are trustworthy. Take reasonable steps to make sure sponsors and partners abide by applicable laws and uphold the same ethical standards.[17]
- Accountability: Provide meaningful opportunity for users to give feedback to the site. Monitor their compliance with the eHealth Code of Ethics.[17]

LEGAL CONSIDERATIONS WITH TELEHEALTH TECHNOLOGY

Federal and state laws govern Telehealth technology and nurses must be compliant to avoid penalties, including sanctions on their registered nurse license. Home health nurses need to review their state's scope of practice law and be aware of Telehealth monitoring crossing outside their state line. It is nurses' responsibility to stay abreast of current laws/policies and any changes that may occur that impact their practice.

National Council of State Boards of Nursing Licensure Issues

The National Council of State Boards of Nursing (NCSBN) closely evaluated the definitions of nursing and the scope of nursing practice with the increasing use of Telehealth technology in patient care. The NCSBN concluded that Telehealth is nursing practice and the regulation of Telehealth nursing is appropriately done by boards of nursing.[18] The NCSBN used home health care nursing as an example of Telehealth nursing practice. NCSBN supported the use of interactive video and technological devices to detect early warning signs of patient complications, document significant changes in a patient condition, and increasing patient access to care.[18]

In response to the expansion of Telehealth nursing across state lines and recognition of Telehealth being an evidence-based model of care delivery, the NCSBN developed a Telehealth policy. In this policy, NCSBN believes that "licensure should be based on the location of the patient as dictated by current law" and "moving licensure to the site of the provider will create confusion for nurses, patients and boards of nursing, not to mention the fact that it will be in direct conflict with states' constitutional rights."[19(p1)] The NCSBN recognized that concerns about licensure was a barrier.

American Telemedicine Association

In May 2014, the American Telemedicine Association updated their Core Standards for Telemedicine Operations.[20] These core standards address guidelines, such as education for the patient, language, privacy, security, confidentiality, mandatory reporting, technical issues including failure, collaborative partnerships, legal and regulatory requirements, jurisdictional regulations, licensing, credentialing, malpractice, and insurance laws.[20] These core standards can be found at their Web site, located at http://www.americantelemed.org/.

Food and Drug Administration Regulation of Mobile Health Technology

There are more than 100,000 Mobile Health (mHealth) applications for medical purposes available to download on portable devices such as smartphones and tablets.[21] Benefits of mHealth are improvement of the quality of medical care, decreased office visits for chronic illnesses, and access to care for patients who are unable or unwilling to attend office visits.[21] In April 2014, new regulations were issued by the Food and Drug Administration (FDA). The FDA will continue to review and approve all new application requests. They also will continue to regulate mHealth apps acting as medical devices to help prevent ineffective and unsafe applications.[21]

FACILITATORS AND BARRIERS TO ADOPTION OF TELEHEALTH TECHNOLOGY

Foster and Sethares[22] investigated what were the facilitators to adoption of Telehealth technology. They also investigated what were the barriers to Telehealth adoption and compliance in the integrative review.[22] The facilitators in the integrative review include the following:

- Devices that have few buttons. Older adults may have decreased cognition and psychomotor skills.
- Automatic transmission of data. A device that is capable of multiple physiologic and mental health data simultaneously requires less time and interference with their lifestyle.
- Low-tech platforms, such as telephones. This can decrease anxiety with learning and is a familiar platform. Learning is easier and empowers self-management.

- Devices that generate reminders or alerts. This will increase compliance and accommodates possible cognitive impairment.
- Both visual and audio guidance. This will provide an alternative learning style to accommodate learning needs.
- User-friendly images appropriate for the older adult. Simple images accommodate visual and perceptual impairment.[22]

Barriers to Telehealth adoption and compliance found in the integrative review include the following[22]:

- Small font is challenging to read.
- Bland graphics and poor contrast is challenging to see and interpret information.
- Devices with widgets are challenging because of poor psychomotor skills with arthritic hands.
- Lack of skill with smartphones and computers can be challenging with cognitive and memory impairment. It can be overwhelming to learn new technological skills.
- Multiple screen transitions to complete a task is too complex to master.
- Menu bars that contain layers of links is complex and overwhelming to learn.
- Smartphone too large or too small making it difficult to grasp.
- Cultural change with learning new technology and not in comfort zone.
- Technical problem and delayed feedback can be frustrating and reduce motivation.[22]

TELEHEALTH IMPACT ON THE HOME HEALTH NURSE'S ROLE

Telehealth has transformed the role of the home health nurse. Telehealth is defined as "the electronic provision of health care and information services for the direct benefit of individual patients and their families."[8(p2)] Technology empowers nurses to increase their patient load, and provide quality, accountable, and safe care. Changes in their role include the following[8]:

- Reduction in documentation: User-friendly software is streamlining forms and providing templates to reduce documentation time, thereby allowing more time with the patient.
- Access to information: Electronic access to patient medical record with diagnostic test results and previous documentation notes.
- Technological support for decision making: Informed decision making with access to decision support systems, monitoring devices, and 2-way video conferencing to provide data for triaging patients. Nurse can text or e-mail physician for quick response for new physician orders.
- Internet Web sites for education materials, and collaborative care via technology tools.[8]

APPLICATION OF TELEHEALTH IN MENTAL HEALTH HOMECARE
Telehealth as Adjunct Therapy for Mental Health

Technologies are available to be used by mental health patients or substance use disorders for self-monitoring and can serve as adjuncts to services provided by professionals. The smart phone app, T2 Mood Tracker, has preloaded scales to be used to track moods. Notes can be entered about medication changes or stressors. Graphs are displayed to track mood changes. This information can be shared with the treatment provider or home health nurse.[23] The PTSD Coach app developed by the

Department of Veterans Affairs allows patients to enter data on experiences and feelings. The app responds with suggested actions, including hotline numbers based on data. The Tactical Breather app is designed to provide management to panic or anxiety reactions. The app uses guided breathing exercises to assist users to control their responses to stress.[23]

Virtual Mental Health Care

E-therapy is the use of technology and communication in any geographic location. It can be used to provide assessment, diagnosis, education, and engagement treatment. Online counseling can be provided to rural areas and underserved areas. E-therapy services can be found in home health care settings, community mental health centers, and military programs.[1] Rating scales are available via computer for the assessment of many mental health disorders, such as depression, anxiety, obsessive-compulsive disorder, and social phobia. These computer-based assessment tools are inexpensive, time-efficient, and a reliable way of assessing symptoms, implementing treatment guidelines, and providing care.[1]

Virtual Reality Technology

Virtual reality creates a real-world environment and can be used for assessment and treatment. This technology can be used for cognitive training and remediation as discussed in the following sections.

Virtual reality functional capacity assessment tool

The virtual reality functional capacity assessment tool (VEFCAT) is a computer-based virtual reality measure of functional capacity consisting of a tutorial and 6 versions of 4 mini scenarios. Patients progress through scenarios, such as navigating a kitchen, catching a bus to a grocery store, and finding/purchasing food in a grocery store. Scores detect impairments and sensitivity to treatment. This program has been used in assessment of elderly and severely mentally ill patients to develop a treatment program to be maintained in the community.[24]

Virtual reality exposure therapy

Exposure therapy is delivered in a real-world environment for treatment of posttraumatic stress disorder. Virtual reality therapy is used to help patients cope with stressful events. Patients are exposed to these events via virtual reality to practice applying coping skills learned in therapy.[25]

Videoconferencing for Disabled Veterans

The program began in 2000 for medication management for veterans disabled or living in rural areas. Videoconferencing has grown to include suicide prevention. In a research study, videoconferencing was found to reduce hospitalization by 24% and the number of days the veterans were hospitalized decreased by 27%.[26]

Internet and E-therapy

E-therapy is the use of the Internet and related media for clinical care. Advances in technology offer communication tools that mental health professionals and patients feel comfortable using for clinical care. Mobile phones are one of the most widespread technologies. Mobile phones have gone from being rare and expensive to low-cost personal items. With the increased usage of mobile telephones, the phone has become a key social and cultural tool.[27] The common use of mobile phones enhances patients' acceptance of its application in mental health education and treatment.[27]

Internet-based resources provide information about health information and support sites. Some sites are more evidence-based than others. It is important for nurses to assess Internet-based resources for credibility and provide patients with appropriate Web sites to find evidence-based information and support for their specific diagnosis.[23]

Chronic Illness Comorbidity with Mental Health Disorders

Mental health patients experience at least one chronic illness that requires monitoring and some degree of self-management. Patients need to be empowered to remain in the home setting by symptom monitoring, compliance to their treatment program, and by having home health nursing support. The use of Telehealth technology can be used for both mental health and chronic illness management by the home health nurse.

CHRONIC ILLNESS

Home Telehealth can be used for management of chronic health problems such as asthma, cardiac disease, diabetes, heart failure, and smoking cessation.[7] The home telephone line provides adequate bandwidth for video telephony, transmission of electrocardiographs, blood pressures, and blood glucose levels, as well as access to the Internet for counseling or education.[7] Retinopathy screening can be done via a retinal camera for diabetic patients in a rural area. The trained nurse can take images and send them by e-mail to an ophthalmologist for evaluation and diagnosis.[7] Tele-radiology can be used to provide radiology services. Portable equipment can be brought to the home to provide radiology services with radiographic images electronically transferred via e-mail from one location to another.[7]

Foster and Sethares[22] conducted an integrative review to determine current Telehealth devices that are used in older adults with chronic illness and what factors are facilitators or barriers to adoption of Telehealth technologies. They found the following Telehealth devices used for older adults with chronic illness in the home setting.[22]

- CoaguChek device was used to determine the international normalized ratios of patients on warfarin (Coumadin). A small droplet of blood from a fingerstick is used to determine a numerical reading that patients enter into a secure Web site on a personal computer. A nurse can respond to the patient via the secure Web site indicating the next warfarin (Coumadin) dose. This device is similar to a blood glucose meter.[22]
- The multiuser Telehealth kiosk system located in an assistive-living home setting allows the resident to insert a personal identification card into the kiosk system. This system allows residents to assess physiologic data, such as blood pressure, heart weight, pulse oximetry, weight, and blood glucose. Collected data are automatically transmitted for analysis.[22]
- The Health Buddy device is an interactive communication device that is attached to a home telephone line that automatically dials a number to upload patients' responses. The program presents questions related to symptoms and information on its screen.[22]
- The American Telecare home telemedicine is a computer system that connects to the Internet over home telephone lines. Patients can send their blood pressure reading and fingerstick glucose values to a health care provider and initiate a video chat to obtain information for self-management.[22]
- The photographic foot imaging device is a computer device composed of a camera module, light source, mirror, glass plate, and foot support to take pictures of diabetic patients' feet. The images are transmitted over the Internet to a secure

provider's office for feet assessment for ulcers or other potential diabetic problems.[22]

- The autotitrating positive airway pressure machine is a modem attached to a home continuous positive airway pressure (CAP) device. This modem can transmit physiologic data such as air leaks, residual apnea-hypopnea index, and CAP adherence for sleep apnea via a telephone line to a Web database for evaluation and adjusts to care if needed.[22]
- A modified bathroom scale with 4 force sensors to evaluate balance and calculate the weight of the patient. A Bluetooth component communicates data via a mobile phone or computer to a remote server for evaluation.[22]
- Smart phone devices allow patients with various medical conditions and mental health problems to access a daily Web-based diary to document their diet, medication compliance, physical activities, emotions, blood pressures, heart rates, and blood glucose from the glucometer. Audio files can be assessed for relaxation and mindfulness exercises.[22]

ELECTRONIC PERSONAL HEALTH RECORDS

There is a growing trend to offer patients access to their personal health records through the use of a patient portal. These records can empower patients in self-management of their health and chronic illnesses. Personalized care plans, graphing of symptoms, diagnoses, diagnostic test results reminders, and motivational feedback can be obtained.[27] The value of electronic personal health records is influenced by its acceptability and usability.[27] Patients need an adequate level of health literacy to be engaged. Research has shown that patients with lower health literacy levels lack the ability to make effective use of Telehealth, have poorer adherence to medical instructions, and are less successful in self-management.[27] Research also shows that lower health literacy levels are particularly prevalent among those with lower levels of educational attainment, those who have a chronic disease or mental illness, and in those older than 65.[27] Home health nurses can assess patient health literacy and help individualize an electronic personal health record to each patient's literacy level.[27] Nurses can help develop a good match to empower patients in self-management of their chronic illness with an electronic personal health record.[27]

SUMMARY

Telehealth technology is an evidence-based delivery model tool that can be integrated into the plan of care for mental health patients. Telehealth technology empowers access to health care, can prevent hospital readmissions, help home health nurses provide shared decision making, and focuses on collaborative care. Telehealth and the recovery model have transformed the role of the home health nurse and increased the quality of patients' lives.

Nurses need to respond to emerging technology and provide cutting-edge evidence-based care. Healthy People 2020 suggests that health communication and information technology can improve population health outcomes, health care quality, and support shared decision making between patients and providers.[4] The 2010 Institute of Medicine Report, *The Future of Nursing*, suggests that nurses need to master technological tools and information systems while collaborating care across interdisciplinary teams.[4] Home health nurses need to develop a nursing skill set of being able to use technology to facilitate mobility, communication, and relationships.[4] Nurses need to develop skills for technology, such as Telehealth, text messaging, videoconferencing, smart phones, social media networking, and embedded sensor networks.[4]

Nurses need to be proactive and respond to rapidly emerging technologies that are transforming the role of home health nurses. Nurses must respond by developing skill competencies for emerging technology to provide safe, quality, and accountable nursing practice to meet positive patient outcomes.

REFERENCES

1. Morrison-Valfre M. Current mental health care systems. Foundations of mental health care. 5th edition. St Louis (MO): Mosby; 2013. p. 10–9 VitalBook file.
2. Halter MJ. Settings for psychiatric care. In: Vararolis EM, editor. Essentials of psychiatric mental health nursing - revised reprint. 2nd edition. St Louis (MO): Saunders; 2014. p. 67–78 VitalBook file.
3. Alper E, O Malley T, Greenwald J. Hospital discharge and readmission. In: Aronson M, Park, editors. p. 1–16. Available at: www.uptodate.com/store. Accessed December 5, 2014.
4. Huston C. The impact of emerging technology on nursing care: warp speed ahead. Online J Issues Nurs 2013;18:1–14.
5. Mohr DC, Schueller SM, Montague E, et al. The behavioral intervention technology model: an integrated conceptual and technological framework for eHealth and mHealth interventions. J Med Internet Res 2014;16(6):146. Available at: https://pod51042.outlook.com/0wa/. Accessed November 24, 2014.
6. President's New Freedom Commission on Mental Health. Achieving the promise: transforming mental health care in America. National Alliance on Mental Illness. Available at: http://www.nami.org. Accessed November 24, 2014.
7. Smith AC, Bensink M, Armfield N, et al. Telemedicine and rural health care applications. J Postgrad Med 2005;51:286–93.
8. Russo H. Window of opportunity for home care nurses: telehealth technologies. Online J Issues Nurs 2001;6(3):5. Available at: www.nursingworld.org/MainMenuCategories/ANAMarketplace/ANAPeriodicals/OJIN/TableofContents/Volume62001/No3Sept01/TelehealthTechnologies.aspx. Accessed November 24, 2014.
9. Choi NG, Hegel MT, Marti NC, et al. Telehealth problem-solving therapy for depressed low-income homebound older adults. Am J Geriatr Psychiatry 2014;22(3):263–71. Available at: http://dx.doi.org/10.1016/j.jagp.2013.01.037. Accessed November 24, 2014.
10. Wenze SJ, Armey MF, Miller IW. Feasibility and acceptability of a mobile intervention to improve treatment adherence in bipolar disorder: a pilot study. Behav Modif 2014;38(4):497–515. Available at: http://www.ncbi.nlm.nih.gov/pubmed/24402464. Accessed November 24, 2014.
11. Taylor J, Coates E, Brewster L, et al. Examining the use of telehealth in community nursing: identifying the factors affecting frontline staff acceptance and telehealth adoption. J Adv Nurs 2015;71(2):326–37. Available at: http://www.pubfacts.com/fulltext_frame.php?PMID=25069605&title=Examining the use of telehealth in community nursing: identifying the factors affecting frontline staff acceptance and telehealth adoption. Accessed November 24, 2014.
12. Lillibridge J, Hanna B. Using telehealth to deliver nursing case management services to HIV/AIDS clients. Online J Issues Nurs 2008;14. Available at: http://dx.doi.org/10.3912/OJIN.Vol14No1PPT02. Accessed November 22, 2014.
13. Bruce ML, Raue PJ, Reill CF, et al. Clinical effectiveness of integrating depression care management into Medicare home health: the depression CAREPATH Randomized Trial. JAMA Intern Med 2015;175(1):55–64.

14. King VL, Brooner RK, Peirce JM, et al. A randomized trial of web-based videocon-ferencing for substance abuse counseling. J Subst Abuse Treat 2014;46(1): 36–42.
15. Seko Y, Kidd S, Wiljer D, et al. Youth mental health interventions via mobile phones: a scoping review. Cyberpsychol Behav Soc Netw 2014;17(9):591–602.
16. Harvey PD, Keefe RS. Technology, society, and mental illness: challenges and opportunities for assessment and treatment. Innov Clin Neurosci 2012; 9(11–12):47–50.
17. Rippen H, Risk A. eHealth code of ethics. J Med Internet Res 2000;2(2):e9. Available at: http://dx.doi.org/10.2196/jmir.2.2e9. Accessed November 24, 2014.
18. National Council of State Boards of Nursing. The National Council of State Boards of Nursing (NCSBN) Position Paper on Telehealth Nursing Practice. 2014. Available at: https://www.ncsbn.org/14_Telehealth.pdf. Accessed November 22, 2014.
19. National Council of State Boards of Nursing. State-based Nursing Licensure and Telehealth. 2014. Available at: https://www.ncsbn.org/LicensureandTelehealth-2014_06.pdf. Accessed November 22, 2014.
20. American Telehealth Association (May 2014) Core Operational Guidelines for Telehealth Services Involving Provider-Patient Interactions. Available at: http://www.americantelemed.org/docs/default-source/standards/core-operational-guidelines-for-telehealth-services.pdf?sfvrsn=6.
21. Cotez NG, Cohen I, Kesselheim AS. FDA regulation of mobile health technology. N Engl J Med 2014;371:372–9. Available at: http://dx.doi.org/10.1056/NEJMhle1403384. Accessed November 22, 2014.
22. Foster MV, Sethares KA. Facilitators and barriers to the adoption of telehealth in older adults: an integrative review. Comput Inform Nurs 2014;32(11):523–33. Available at: http://dx.doi.org/10.1097/CIN.000000000000.105. Accessed November 22, 2014.
23. Lauerman V. Using technology as an adjunct therapy for mental health treatment. Doral Health. Available at: http://www.dorlandhealth.com/dorland-health-articles/CIP_0113_24_Techxml. Accessed November 24, 2014.
24. Ruse SA, Harvey PD, Davis VG, et al. Virtual reality capacity assessment in schizophrenia: preliminary data regarding feasibility and correlations with cognitive and functional capacity performance. Schizophr Res Cogn 2014;1(1):e21–6. Available at: http://www.ncbi.nlm.nih.gov/pubmed/25083416. Accessed November 30, 2014.
25. Prexiosa A, Grassi A, Gaggioli A, et al. Therapeutic applications of the mobile phone. Br J Guid Counc 2009;37(3):313–25.
26. US Department of Veterans Affairs Veterans Health Administration. Using technology to improve access to mental health care. Available at: http://www.va.gov/health/NewsFeatures/20120813a.asp. Accessed November 22, 2014.
27. Mitchell B, Begoray D. Electronic personal health records that promote self-management in chronic illness. Online J Issues Nurs 2010;15(3). Available at: http://dx.doi.org/10.3912/OJIN.Vol15No03PPT01. Accessed November 22, 2014.

Potentials of Internet-Based Patient Engagement and Education Programs to Reduce Hospital Readmissions
A Spotlight on Need in Heart Failure

Christian Ketel, DNP, RN

KEYWORDS

- Internet-based platforms/applications • M-health • Patient engagement
- Care-management • Readmission avoidance • Heart failure • Self-management

KEY POINTS

- The most prominent example and precursor to this technology is the patient portal.
- Internet-based (IB) applications range in functionality and scope from readily available and unmonitored Internet sites providing health information to highly regulated and protected patient care online environments, such as patient portals and telemedicine applications.
- IB applications and mobile technologies (m-Health) are becoming an attractive platform for readmission avoidance programs for patients with heart failure, and for other conditions at high risk for readmission.

INTRODUCTION

Treatment of heart failure (HF) largely depends on the ability of patients to engage in effective self-management activities. The Heart Failure Society of America (HFSA) provides comprehensive guidelines for the education of both HF patients and their caregivers. The essential elements of an HF program are based on targeted behaviors that focus on the following elements: (1) understanding of the overall disease process, (2) recognition of symptoms, (3) indications for medications, (4) modification of risks for disease progression, (5) specific activity and exercise recommendations, and (6) importance of adherence to treatment plan.[1]

Largely based on these elements, hospital-based readmission reduction programs are becoming standard throughout the United States. This increased interest in reducing readmission is at least partially motivated by the threat of financial penalties for excessive

Clinical Practice and Community Partnerships, Vanderbilt University School of Nursing, 1024-C 18th Avenue South, Nashville, TN 37212, USA
E-mail address: Christian.Ketel@vanderbilt.edu

Nurs Clin N Am 50 (2015) 283–291
http://dx.doi.org/10.1016/j.cnur.2015.02.003 nursing.theclinics.com
0029-6465/15/$ – see front matter © 2015 Elsevier Inc. All rights reserved.

readmission, but is also motivated by the organization's wish to improve the health and quality of life of the individuals and families in the communities they serve.[2] In addition to hospitals taking notice of the financial ramifications associated with reducing readmissions, insurance companies are also developing strategies to reduce readmissions for their beneficiaries.[3] In most cases, hospitals and insurance providers are using programs that are primarily focused on increasing postdischarge contact with the patient through home visits and via the telephone. The secondary focus of these programs is to improve self-management behaviors through disease-specific education and support for patients and caregivers.[4–6] In light of these factors and motivations, hospitals have become open to trialing innovative and cost-effective strategies to both reduce readmission rates and improve patient outcomes. Specifically, HF contributes to more than 1 million hospital admissions each year, costing the American population more than $20 billion annually. When direct and indirect costs of HF are assessed, the costs are astronomical. It is estimated that those costs exceeded $40 billion in 2010 with costs expected to increase.[7] To mitigate or counter this expected increase in readmission, affordable and easily scalable Internet-based (IB) strategies are becoming increasingly attractive to any organizations that either are responsible for paying for potentially avoidable hospitalizations (insurance companies and accountable care organizations) or that incur stiff penalties for deviations in optimum care (hospitals).

Many of these strategies include the use of health information technology. These technologies are gathering more popularity as potentially viable means of improving care efficiency, patient safety, and patient outcomes. Technological developments such as electronic medical records, computerized medication ordering and prescribing, and decision support are now recognized as making a significant difference in both outpatient and inpatient care.

In general, these improvements are in response to enhanced work flows, improved communication, predictive modeling, and identification and stratification of patient risk.[8] In most of these examples, the focus has been on improving the way that clinicians (nurses, doctors, clinical pharmacists, social workers, and so forth) provide care to the patient. The success of these provider-focused technologies to improve outcomes, in combination with the explosive growth of Internet-based communication capacities, have stimulated considerable thought and energy around developing novel approaches to the traditional provider/patient therapeutic interaction or IB patient engagement and education programs.

The most prominent example and precursor to this technology is the patient portal. The term patient portal implies a variety of software solutions that give both patients and their providers the ability to have a shared view of a patient's health information and the ability to hold a dialogue about that information. The hope is that these technologies will improve communication between the patient and clinician, and shift the ultimate management of individual health toward the patient.[9]

As stated previously, the time between inpatient and outpatient care, termed transitional care, is a time of high risk for patients and families in the postdischarge stage. The use of IB patient engagement strategies is relatively new, but these innovations offer promising potential for improving patient engagement and education, enhancing provider-patient and provider-provider communication, and reducing unnecessary hospital readmission from avoidable causes.[8,10]

HEART FAILURE READMISSIONS: A POTENTIALLY AVOIDABLE SITUATION

HF contributes to 32% to 35% of the hospitalization admissions in the United States each year.[11] Of these patients, approximately 25% are readmitted within 30 days of discharge.[12] HF is an extremely complex disease, and some readmissions may be unavoidable owing to the underlying debilitating nature of the condition. However, it is suggested that most readmissions are attributed to avoidable causes such as medication nonadherence, inadequate social support, and noncompliance to lifestyle modifications.[13] Often the patient is unprepared to deal with the self-management demands associated with HF.[14]

To address this problem, a variety of postdischarge IB education and monitoring programs are currently being developed, with goals including, but not limited to, improving patient self-efficacy and reducing hospital readmission for HF patients.[15]

HEART FAILURE DEFINED

HF is defined as a loss or dysfunction of the myocardium as a result of elevated cardiac filling pressures or inadequate peripheral oxygen delivery, primarily characterized by left ventricular dilation or hypertrophy.[16,17] Once the process of dysfunction is set in motion from varied systolic or diastolic causes, HF is generally progressive and fatal. The primary causes of HF are myocardial infarction, coronary artery disease, longstanding hypertension, valvular disease, myocardial infection, and as a side effect of some medications (eg, cancer chemotherapeutic agents).[7] Other than heart transplantation, there are few instances whereby HF progression can be stopped or reversed once it is set into motion. However, with sustained lifestyle modification and adherence to HF management therapy, patients can drastically slow the progression of the disease, have therapeutically induced improvements in cardiac function, and experience an overall decrease in HF symptoms.[7]

FACTORS CONTRIBUTING TO HOSPITAL READMISSION FOR HEART FAILURE

Chun and colleagues[18] followed more than 8000 patients with HF over the course of their lifetime from the time of their first hospital admission. It was established that greater than 30% of the HF patients in the study were readmitted to hospital within 30 days of discharge and that more than 66% were admitted within 1 year. It is well established that nonadherence to treatment regimens is a leading cause of worsening HF, and places patients at an increased risk for hospitalization and readmissions.[19–21]

The risk for readmission and the necessity to avoid it are not new concepts to hospital administrators or accountable care organizations, but both have gained increasingly more attention as the structure of hospital readmission reimbursement has tightened and the monetary penalties for readmission are now a distinct reality. These changes are in large part due to the Readmission Reduction Program initiated by the Centers for Medicare and Medicaid Services to levy large penalties for hospitals that have moderate to high levels of 30-day readmission rates.[22] Readmission avoidance programs that are aimed at reducing the 30-day readmission are being widely implemented, and the use of information technology solutions are of great interest because of their potential to be both clinically and cost effective.[23]

SELF-EFFICACY AND SELF-MANAGEMENT: A POTENTIAL SOLUTION

Barlow and colleagues[24(p178)] summed it up well by defining self-management as "the individual's ability to manage the symptoms, treatment, physical and social consequences, and lifestyle changes inherent in living with a chronic condition." This approach is easily applied to a variety of chronic diseases, such as diabetes, asthma, renal disease, and the primary focus of this article, HF (**Box 1**).

> **Box 1**
> **Five components of a successful self-management**
>
> - Participating in decision making
> - Building sustained health relationships
> - Monitoring and managing symptoms
> - The ability to acquire knowledge and leverage resources
> - The ability to develop and execute a plan of action
>
> *Data from* Lorig K, Holman H. Self-management education: history, definition, outcomes, and mechanisms. Ann Behav Med 2003;26(1):1–7.

By comparison, self-efficacy is defined as the belief in oneself that one can perform a desired task or achieve a desired outcome.[25] Although these 2 concepts appear identical on the surface, they may be better viewed as corresponding parts of the larger, broader concept of self-care. Self-efficacy is best described as an outcome or result of the combined activities involved in self-management.

Self-management programs are designed to facilitate the ability of patients to make informed choices, learn problem-solving skills, practice new health behaviors, and maintain emotional stability.[26] Self-management is aimed at improving health status and slowing the progressive deterioration associated with chronic disease, such as HF. A potential outcome of effective self-management is reduction in the need for health care services. Overall, self-management activities are intended to help patients become active partners in their own health care.

HF patients, in particular, must participate in self-management to maintain a delicate balance between optimal health and symptomatic heart failure.[7] Self-management of HF involves cognitive decision making in response to signs and symptoms of HF exacerbation. Because the greater part of HF care takes place at home, it is important for individuals with HF and their caregivers to understand their condition and treatment.[19]

INTERNET-BASED APPLICATIONS AND MOBILE TECHNOLOGY: THE MEDIATOR

IB applications and mobile technologies (m-health) are becoming an attractive platform for readmission avoidance programs for patients with HF and for other conditions at high risk for readmission. IB applications represent a wide range of electronic services or programs that are commonly referred to as "Software as a Service" (SaaS). SaaS programs are generally accessed through a Web browser via the Internet, and data generated are stored in a centrally located electronic data repositories often referred to as the cloud.[27] IB applications encompass m-health technologies. M-Health can be defined as "the use of mobile devices to communicate [or exchange] health information."[28(p1)]

Technological precursors or forerunners to both IB applications and m-health programs being used in health care currently are telephone monitoring and short message service (SMS) texting technology. A study by Nundy and colleagues[29] provides a good example of the use of SMS texting. In this study, African American participants being treated for heart failure were sent daily text reminders with topics including medications use, diet, appointment adherence, signs and symptoms of exacerbation, and health navigation. Both telephone monitoring and SMS texting technology have had mixed but predominately favorable results in influencing the health of patients.[30] Building off these technologies, IB applications and m-health technologies both take advantage of society's increasing interest in technology and engagement with the online environment.[31] IB applications range in functionality and scope from readily available and unmonitored Internet sites providing health information to highly regulated and protected patient care online environments, such as patient portals and telemedicine applications.

Both telephone and secure messaging patient engagement have been shown to be as effective as in-person education for chronic disease states such as diabetes.[32] Email via Web-based interaction between patient and provider is the newest engagement strategy being currently evaluated, largely because of the higher prevalence of Internet connectivity and the wider availability and affordability of Internet-capable devices such as desktop computers, laptops, and various tablets and smartphones.[33] A recent feasibility study examining the use of Internet-based technology in the management of chronic disease identified that Internet access or device availability was not a significant barrier. However, disease burden and information technology literacy were found to pose the greatest barriers to the application.[34]

SIGNIFICANCE TO HEALTH CARE

HF contributes to well in excess of 1 million hospital admissions each year, costing the American population more than $20 billion annually. When direct and indirect costs of HF assessed, the costs are astronomical. It is estimated that such costs exceeded $40 billion in 2010, with an expected increase in years to come.[7]

IB applications incorporating m-health technology have been investigated in other chronic disease states. Diabetes, in particular, is a disease that has been shown to be amenable to programs using m-health technologies. The World Health Organization defines m-health broadly as medical and public health practices that incorporate mobile devices, such as cellular smartphones, patient monitoring devices, personal digital assistants, and other wireless devices.[35] In a pilot study evaluating an m-health–based diabetes self-management program performed by Katz and colleagues,[36] researchers reported increases in disease self-management behaviors and improvements in hemoglobin A1c (HbA1c) levels in participants who were active in the program. Participants who did not engage with the program showed minimal increases in self-management behaviors and HbA1c levels.

The engagement rates with the program in this study were higher than 60%, which raises the question of whether barriers to engagement have an influence overall on programs based on IB application and m-health technology. In a larger, more disease-diverse retrospective study of more than 1000 chronically ill veterans, participants were asked to engage in an automated self-management patient monitor telephone call system. In this population, 71% of the calls to participants were answered.[37] These findings lend support to the potential use of IB applications and m-health technologies in the treatment of chronic disease. More specifically, they support the use of these technologies in the management of HF.[30]

DISCUSSION

Treatment modalities, both pharmacologic and nonpharmacologic, are well studied and well established. It has been shown that an adherence to medication, diet, and lifestyle changes leads to decreases in morbidity and mortality and an increase in overall quality of life.[21] The literature, however, is not as convincing regarding the optimal way to achieve adequate adherence to the complex requirements of an HF program in the home or an outpatient setting.[38] Achieving the sustained lifestyle modification necessary for long-term adherence to lifestyle modification continues to be a challenge. It does seem apparent that regular and frequent contact between a patient and a health care provider offers the highest levels of success.[6,7]

Weaknesses arise when considering the current evidence supporting the use of IB application or m-health technology to improve self-management behaviors and overall self-efficacy. The first major weakness is the propensity for studies to focus on highly educated, white participants.[39–42] This selection bias leads to difficulty in applying the evidence to more diverse populations. The second weakness is that most programs based on IB application and m-health technology have at best shown adherence rates of 60% to 75%.[37,43] This level of engagement may not prove to have enough of an impact to justify the costs of IB application and m-health innovations. The last major weakness concerns the small study size and correspondingly low sample size of the studies published to date.[44] This situation will likely be nullified in the near future by the high level of interest in the use of IB applications and m-health technologies by both government and private sector stakeholders.[45]

It is well established that disease self-management activities are critical for the overall success of HF treatment and that self-management activities depend on adequate knowledge. The popularity and growing accessibility of the Internet and the practical implications of IB activities provide a promising alternative for implementing HF programs. More evidence is needed to determine whether IB applications and m-health technologies can have an impact on patient self-management behaviors, as evidenced by increased overall self-efficacy and disease management and decreasing hospital admissions/readmissions for patients with HF.

The use of IB and mobile technology tools and programs by nurses and patients will be necessary to meet the demands of the increasing responsibility of hospitals to prevent and reduce 30-day readmissions in view of increasing patient numbers and acuity. There continue to be a variety of identified and unidentified barriers keeping clinician teams, including nursing, from enrolling patients and patients from engaging with the desired technology. These barriers need to be evaluated much further to determine and inform the further development of IB and mobile technologies, particularly among the lower-income, non-Caucasian patient populations. These technological tools have the potential to support patients of all diagnoses throughout the early recovery period after hospital admission and to prevent unnecessary readmission through increased self-management behaviors. More importantly, they provide better communication in a time of turbulent change between the health care community and the patients they serve.

ACKNOWLEDGMENTS

I would like to acknowledge Patricia Trangenstein, PhD, RN-BC; Catherine Ivory, PhD; and Bonnie Pilon, PhD, NEA-BC, FAAN for their support through my Doctor from Nursing Practice Capstone Process from which much of this article is based. Specifically, I would like to thank each of them for their ongoing mentorship and expert guidance.

REFERENCES

1. Lindenfeld J, Albert N, Boehmer J, et al. HFSA 2010 comprehensive heart failure practice guidelines. J Card Fail 2010;16:e1–194.
2. Kansagara D, Englander H, Salanitro A, et al. Risk prediction models for hospital readmission: a systematic review. JAMA 2011;306(15):1688–98.

3. Bayer E. An update on health plan initiatives to address national health care priorities. Washington, DC: American's Health Insurance Plans, Center for Policy and Research; 2010.

4. Jack B, Chetty V, Anthony D, et al. A reengineered hospital discharge program to decrease rehospitalization. Ann Intern Med 2009;150(3):178–87.

5. Coleman E, Parry C, Chalmers S, et al. The care transitions intervention: results of a randomized controlled trial. Arch Intern Med 2006;166:1822–8.

6. Phillip C, Wright S, Kern D, et al. Comprehensive discharge planning with postdischarge support for older patients with congestive heart failure: a meta-analysis. JAMA 2004;291(11):1358–67.

7. Yancy C, Bozkurt J, Masaudi F, et al. 2013 ACCF/AHA Guideline for the management of heart failure. J Am Coll Cardiol 2013;62:e146–239.

8. Institute of Medicine of the National Academies. Health IT and patient safety: building safer systems for better care. Washington, DC: National Academies Press; 2012. p. 1–12.

9. Palen T, Bayliss E, Steiner J. Are patient portals on key to unlocking the door for engaging patients in their healthcare? J Comp Eff Res 2013;2:99–101.

10. HIMSS. Reducing readmissions: top ways information technology can help. Chicago: 2012. Available at: http://www.himss.org/files/HIMSSorg/content/files/ControlReadmissionsTechnology.pdf. Accessed April 11, 2013.

11. CDC. Hospitalizations for congestive heart failure. 2012. Available at: http://www.cdc.gov/nchs/data/databriefs/db108.htm. Accessed November 2, 2013.

12. HHS. All cause 30-day readmission rates after hospitalization with congestive heart failure. 2012. Available at: https://healthmeasures.aspe.hhs.gov/measure/8a. Accessed November 12, 2013.

13. Inglis S, Clark A, McAlister F, et al. Structured telephone support or telemonitoring programmes for patients with chronic heart failure. Cochrane Database Systems Review 2010;8:1–138.

14. Meyers A, Salanitro A, Wallston K, et al. Determinants of heath after hospital discharge: rationale and design of the Vanderbilt Inpatient Cohort Study (VICS). BMC Health Serv Res 2014;14:1–10.

15. Klersy C, Silvestri A, Gabutti G, et al. A meta-analysis of remote monitoring of heart failure patients. J Am Coll Cardiol 2009;54(18):1683–94.

16. American Heart Association. What is heart failure? 2012. Available at: http://www.heart.org/idc/groups/heart-public/@wcm/@hcm/documents/downloadable/ucm_300315.pdf. Accessed April 11, 2013.

17. Go A, Mozaffarian D, Rogers V, et al. Heart disease and stroke statistics-2013 update from the American Heart Association. Circulation 2014;127:e6–245.

18. Chun S, Tu J, Wijjeysundrea H, et al. Lifetime analysis of hospitalizations and survival of patients newly admitted with heart failure. Circ Heart Fail 2012;5:414–21.

19. Adams K, Lindenfeld J, Arnold J, et al. Executive summary: Heart Failure Society of America 2006 comprehensive heart failure practice guidelines. J Card Fail 2006;12:10–38.

20. Tsuyuki R, Fradette M, Johnson J, et al. A multicenter disease management program for hospitalized patients with heart failure. J Cardiol 2004;10(6):473–80.

21. Butler J, Kalogeropoulos A. Hospital strategies to reduce heart failure: where is the evidence. J Am Coll Cardiol 2012;60:615–7.

22. Centers for Medicare and Medicaid Services. Readmission reduction program. 2013. Available at: http://www.cms.gov/Medicare/Medicare-Fee-for-Service-Payment/AcuteInpatientPPS/Readmissions-Reduction-Program.html. Accessed November 1, 2013.

23. Hines S. Reducing avoidable hospital readmissions. Health Research and Educational Trust. Rockvale (MD): Agency for Healthcare Research and Quality; 2011. Available at: http://www.ahrq.gov/news/kt/red/readmissionslides/readslide5.htm.

24. Barlow J, Wright C, Sheasby J, et al. Self- management approaches for people with chronic conditions: a review. Patient Educ Couns 2002;48(2):177–87.

25. Bandura A. Social foundations of thought and action. Englewood Cliffs (NJ): Prentice-Hall; 1986.

26. Lorig K, Mazonson P, Holman H. Evidence suggesting that health education for self-management in the chronic arthritis has sustained health benefits while reducing health care costs. Arthritis Rheum 1993;36(4):439–46.

27. JBuilder. Web application developer's guide. Scotts Valley (CA): Borland Software Corporation; 2002.

28. Sherry J, Ratzan S. Measurement and evaluation outcomes for mHealth communication. J Health Commun 2012;17:1–3.

29. Nundy S, Razi R, Dick J, et al. A text messaging intervention to improve heart failure self-management after hospital discharge in a large African-American population: before-after study. J Med Internet Res 2013;15:e53.

30. Shatz T, Ratzan S. The potential of an online and mobile health scorecard for preventing chronic disease. J Health Commun 2013;16:175–90.

31. Maged B, Wheeler S, Tavares C, et al. How smartphones are changing the face of mobile and participatory healthcare: an overview, with example fromCAALYX. Biomed Eng Online 2011;10:24. Available at: http://www-ncbi-nlm-nih-gov.proxy.library.vanderbilt.edu/pmc/articles/PMC3080339/pdf/1475-925X-10-24.pdf.

32. Greenwood D, Hankins A, Parise C, et al. A comparison of in-person, telephone, and secure messaging for type 2 diabetes self-management support. Diabetes Educ 2014;40(4):516–25.

33. Hung M, Conrad J, Hon S, et al. Uncovering patterns of technology use in consumer health informatics. Wiley Interdiscip Rev Comput Stat 2013;5(6):432–47.

34. Schrader G, Bidargaddi N, Harris M, et al. An ehealth intervention in rural areas: preliminary findings from a pilot feasibility study. JMIR Res Protoc 2014;13:e27.

35. World Health Organization. mHealth: new horizons for health through mobile technologies. Global observatory for eHealth series, vol. 3. 2011. Available at: http://www.who.int/goe/publications/goe_mhealth_web.pdf. Accessed January 21, 2014.

36. Katz R, Mesfin T, Barr K. Lessons from a community-based mhealth diabetes self-management program: "it's not just about the cell phone". J Health Commun 2012;17:67–72.

37. Piette J, Rosland A, Marcinec N, et al. Engagement with automated patient monitoring and self-management support calls: experience with a thousand chronically ill patients. Med Care 2013;51:216–23.

38. Lorig K, Holman H. Self-management education: history, definition, outcomes, and mechanisms. Ann Behav Med 2003;26(1):1–7.

39. Jackson C, Bolen S, Brancati F, et al. A systematic review of interactive computer-assisted technology in diabetes care. J Gen Intern Med 2006;21:105–10.

40. Lorig K, Ritter P, Laurent D, et al. Online diabetes self-management program: a randomized trial. Diabetes Care 2010;33(6):1275–81.

41. Lorig K, Ritter P, Plant K, et al. Internet-based chronic disease self-management: a randomized trial. Med Care 2006;44(11):964–71.

42. Ross S, Moore L, Earnest M, et al. Providing a web-based online medical record with electronic communication capabilities to patients with congestive heart

failure: randomized trial. J Med Internet Res 2004;6:e2. Available at: http://www.jmir.org.proxy.library.vanderbilt.edu/2004/2/e12/.

43. Lorig K, Ritter P, Laurent D, et al. The internet-based self-management program: a one-year randomized trial for patient with arthritis or fibromyalgia. Arthritis Rheum 2008;15(7):1009–17.

44. Murray E, Burns J, See T, et al. Interactive health communication application for people with chronic disease. Cochrane Database Syst Rev 2005;(4). CD004274. Available   at: http://onlinelibrary.wiley.com.proxy.library.vanderbilt.edu/doi/10.1002/14651858.

45. Avalere Health. Delivering value in healthcare: a multi-stakeholder vision for innovation. Washington, DC: Avalere Health, LLC; 2013.

Nurse Knowledge of Intrahospital Transport

John Shields, DNP, CRNA[a,b,*], Maria Overstreet, PhD, RN[c,d],
Stephen D. Krau, PhD, RN, CNE[d]

KEYWORDS

- Intrahospital transport (IHT) • Patient safety • Clinical handover • Nurse anesthesia
- Nurse

KEY POINTS

- Preventable adverse events and other medical errors occur to hundreds of thousands of Americans every year. The financial burden of these preventable events is estimated to be $29 billion. According to the World Health Organization, reducing medical errors has become an international concern.

- Protecting patients from harm is a primary responsibility of all nurses regardless of whether the nurse works in the intensive care unit or operating room. Adherence to intrahospital transport (IHT) policies to maintain patient safety can be discerned once the level of the knowledge of these policies among nurses is determined.

- Improving patient safety during IHT involves management of essential elements of IHT, including communication, personnel, equipment, and monitoring. Although patient safety obstacles are apparent in each stage of IHT, communication during handover is consistently inadequate. Knowledge of the clinical handover policy is essential in following established structure during communication. Recommendations for improving patient safety during IHT consistently include equipment management, team composition, and enhanced communication through education and training.

- Recognition of IHT risk requires anticipatory guidance and communication between providers. Assembling proper equipment and medications for IHT depend on providers knowing their role based on policies generated by the organization.

- The analysis of survey results also demonstrates differences in 3 core elements of IHT among the provider groups: preplanning, personnel requirements, and communication. Knowledge of these 3 elements and policies differ significantly among providers, whereas no differences exist because of experience with IHT or training. As clinical decision making is based more on best practice and policy, knowledge of policies is essential.

Disclosure: None.

[a] Cardiac Anesthesia Division, Department of Anesthesiology, Vanderbilt University Medical Center, 1301 Medical Center Drive, 4648 TVC, Nashville, TN 37232-5614, USA; [b] Middle Tennessee School of Anesthesia, 315 Hospital Drive, Madison, TN 37115, USA; [c] Center for Clinical Simulation, Middle Tennessee School of Anesthesia, Madison, TN 37115, USA; [d] Vanderbilt School of Nursing, 1301 Medical Center Drive, 4648 TVC, Nashville, TN 37232-5614, USA
* Corresponding author. Middle Tennessee School of Anesthesia, 315 Hospital Drive, Madison, TN 37115.
E-mail address: john.shields@mtsa.edu

NURSE KNOWLEDGE OF INTRAHOSPITAL TRANSPORT: A DOCTORATE OF NURSING PRACTICE PROJECT

Critically ill patients are transferred to locations outside the intensive care unit (ICU) by intrahospital transport (IHT) for procedures or diagnostic testing. Up to 52% of patients in ICUs are transported at least once to departments such as surgery.[1] During these transports, up to 70% of patients may suffer an adverse event, such as hypotension, dysrhythmias, hypoxemia, or cardiac arrest.[2] In 2001, the Agency for Healthcare Research and Quality (AHRQ) recognized these types of IHT to be a patient safety issue and placed priority on development of practices to reduce patient risk (http://archive.ahrq.gov/clinic/ptsafety/chap47.htm). Warren and colleagues[3] developed safety guidelines for IHT components (team composition, handover communication, and checklists) and recommended planning, use of qualified personnel, and focus on proper equipment management. Despite these guidelines and recommendations, adverse events and patient safety issues continue to occur during IHT. In 2007, equipment and patient instability were identified as issues contributing to adverse events, whereas training and education were recommended to improve adherence with guidelines.[4] Adverse events may occur in up to 68% of all IHT, with 4.2% to 8.9% requiring therapeutic interventions.[5]

To transport critically ill patients in a safe and effective manner, a large magnet hospital in the Southeastern United States developed a specific IHT policy and a clinical handover policy, including specific definitions and procedures. The anesthesia department created a checklist describing core elements of IHT for direct admissions and specified equipment and personnel required for IHT. Data from this hospital's perioperative enterprise reporting revealed the main operating room performed 3294 procedures on patients from the trauma ICU (TICU) from January 1, 2012 to June 30, 2012. During this period, approximately 12% or 397 of these patients were transferred directly from the TICU to the operating room using IHT. As adverse events may occur in up to 70% of all IHT, compliance with the hospital's IHT policy is essential in minimizing risk.

The assessment of compliance with IHT policy begins with an evaluation of potential failure modes that may interfere with the implementation of safety policies.[6] The scope of this project included examination of the primary findings from the literature regarding patient safety issues during IHT, description of hospital policies, and checklists for IHT and assessment of ICU nurse and nurse anesthetists' knowledge of these policies. Five core elements of IHT derived from the literature were assessed in this project: (1) preplanning, (2) appropriate personnel, (3) appropriate equipment, (4) continuous monitoring, and (5) documentation/communication of patient status.[7] The results of this project provide insight into provider knowledge, which is foundational to the direction of future quality and patient safety improvement efforts.

STATEMENT OF THE PROBLEM

IHT is associated with adverse events and presents risk for patient safety.[2–5,8] Despite safety initiatives, adverse events continue to occur and can include hypoxemia, hypothermia, arrhythmia, hypotension, hypertension, pneumothorax, intracranial hypertension, accidental extubation/loss of airway, bronchospasm, equipment failure, wrong patient transports, cardiac arrest, and death.[5]

At the hospital that provided the setting for this project, IHT affects 12% of trauma patients undergoing surgery. The hospital has a specific policy for IHT, which includes guidelines for preplanning, equipment, monitoring, personnel, and communication to support the patients' physiologic needs during transport. Steps in the process of IHT are listed in hospital policies and the anesthesia department checklist. These steps include

- The nurse anesthetist reviews the patient status with the anesthesiologist before transport, and the anesthesia team develops a management plan.
- The ICU nurse is called by the nurse anesthetist or student nurse anesthetist, and the report is obtained while the notification of transport is delivered.
- Personnel requirements for transport of mechanically ventilated and unstable patients mandate that at least 3 licensed staff (one of whom is a nurse anesthetist) accompany the patients.
- Criteria established to determine patient stability include continuous use of vasoactive infusions to control blood pressure, use of pulmonary vasodilators, significant metabolic acidosis, persistent hypotension (systolic blood pressure <80 mm Hg), respiratory distress, and unstable airway.
- Monitoring equipment and medications are gathered by the nurse anesthetist before proceeding to the unit.
- The level of monitoring and care during IHT is to be consistent with the patients' prescribed level of care in the ICU.
- Immediately before transport, a nurse anesthetist must receive a structured report or handover from an ICU nurse.
- Communication and handover is to be consistent with clinical handover policy and includes uninterrupted, interactive structured 2-way communication with anticipatory guidance.

Current literature and hospital policy support a framework using 5 core elements for IHT.[7] The hospital that provided the setting for the project addresses these 5 elements in its policies and the checklist. Knowledge of these policies and checklist is essential in limiting adverse events. Potential failure modes involving these elements may include

- Preplanning
  - Lack of coordination between anesthesia and the ICU
- Personnel
  - Inadequate number of staff
  - Inadequate training of staff
  - Inappropriate composition of team
- Equipment
  - Faulty equipment
  - Inadequate equipment
- Monitoring
  - Inadequate monitoring
  - Inadequate level of provider for level of required monitoring
- Communication
  - Inadequate handover
  - Lack of handover training

Training for IHT is not mandated, but the hospital's clinical handover policy states that the clinical staff will receive education and training to perform structured handovers including the use of an organizationally approved structure. The structure used at the project hospital is *SBAR*, which is an acronym for a method of communicating critical information focusing on *situation, background, assessment, and recommendations*. Without knowledge of the policies and handover structure, inconsistent or lack of communication may lead to a higher risk of adverse outcomes. The level of understanding and comprehension of these policies by the hospital's health care providers is unknown.

PURPOSE, AIMS, AND OBJECTIVES

The purpose of this project was to assess nurse knowledge of the procedure for IHT and clinical handover as defined by the hospital's IHT and clinical handover policies. Aims of the project included characterizing IHT team members' knowledge and understanding of core policy components. Specific objectives for this project included assessment of TICU nurse, nurse anesthetist, and student nurse anesthetist's knowledge of IHT and clinical handover policies of the 5 core elements of IHT. IHT procedures as defined by policy include detailed description of preplanning, personnel, equipment, medications, and communication expectations. Preplanning for IHT was assessed in a survey of nurses including specific components, such as patient preparation and communication. Personnel components for IHT were assessed through a survey of team composition and criteria for stability. Knowledge of equipment and supply needs was assessed including functionality, responsibilities of the team, and transport requirements. The communication structure of IHT was assessed through a survey of handover content, format of the communication during handover, and the specific information that was exchanged. Anticipatory guidance including continuing therapies and special patient considerations was assessed along with transition-of-care strategies.

TECHNOLOGY SUPPORT FOR PROJECT

The technology used to support this project was in the form of an Internet survey whereby data were collected and analyzed in a confidential fashion. The method used to send and return surveys was Web based and used the Research Electronic Data Capture (REDCap) survey system and project hospital's e-mail structure. The survey was created using REDCap, which provides an interface for validated data entry, audit trails for tracking data manipulation, automated export procedures for data downloads to statistical packages, as well as import of data from external sources. REDCap is a secure, Web-based application designed to support data capture for research studies. Data can be easily deidentified and exported to common statistical packages, such as Statistical Package for the Social Sciences Version 21 (SPSS). REDCap was selected, as it is a known entity at the project site; assistance is available from the project site in using the application; and it is populated with e-mail addresses of participants. Confidentiality was maintained and anonymity insured through the REDCap secure database.

BACKGROUND

IHT is described by the AHRQ as the "transportation of patients within a hospital for the purpose of undergoing diagnostic or therapeutic procedures or transfer to a specialized unit."[9,10(p534)] The AHRQ recognizes that critically ill patients going to surgery are "at a high risk for complications en route"[9(p534)] and recommend the development of practices to minimize or reduce risk associated with this practice. In an attempt to reduce risk, the project hospital implemented policies and procedures specific to handover behavior and communication as well as the standard procedure for IHT. IHT policy provides guidelines for safe transport to a receiving department or unit, as with IHT from TICU to surgery. Along with hospital policies regarding IHT, the anesthesia department developed a direct transport checklist to mandate strict IHT protocols, including IHT team composition, communication between ICU nurse and nurse anesthetist, equipment requirements, patient identification, and surgical consent verification. Provider to provider handover includes any special patient considerations, and communication is to be consistent with the hospital's clinical handover communication policy. The clinical handover policy provides a structure for this handover, including an interactive two-way communication, uninterrupted attention by the giver and receiver free from other responsibilities and focus on anticipatory guidance. No known visible structure exists for training or education for IHT or clinical handover. The level of knowledge among nurses related to IHT and clinical handover as outlined by the policies is not known. In cases where knowledge or understanding of policies designed to achieve optimal patient outcomes and assure patient safety is unknown, there is tremendous potential for adverse events.

SIGNIFICANCE
Health Care

The potential life and dollar savings from the elimination of adverse events caused by IHT error may be tremendous, and the widespread use of policy and training would increase safety.[5] Preventable adverse events and other medical errors occur to hundreds of thousands of Americans every year.[11] The financial burden of these preventable events is estimated to be $29 billion.[12] According to the World Health Organization, reducing medical errors has become an international concern (http://www.who.int/patientsafety/events//05/Reporting_Guidelines.pdf). The Centers for Disease Control and Prevention affirms if preventable medical error was listed as a disease process it would be the sixth leading cause of death in the United States (www.cdc.gov/nchs/fastats/deaths.htm).

Patient safety and avoiding inadvertent harm from error came to the forefront of patient care based on the Institute of Medicine's (IOM) report *To Err is Human* (2000).[11] Adverse events associated with IHT persist; McLenon[13] classifies them into 2 categories: patient-based and systems-based errors. IHT policy has been developed at this hospital to avoid issues such as communication errors, equipment malfunction and anticipation of physiologic deterioration through preplanning, adequate personnel and equipment, maintenance of the same level of monitoring, and communication.

Nursing

Transport of critically ill patients from the ICU to the operating room is a necessary part of patient care. Protecting patients from harm is a primary responsibility of all nurses regardless of whether the nurse works in the ICU or operating room. Adherence to policies to maintain patient safety can only be discerned once the level of the knowledge of these policies among nurses is determined. Improving patient safety during IHT involves management of essential elements of IHT, including communication, personnel, equipment, and monitoring.[3] Although patient safety obstacles are apparent in each stage of IHT, Ong and Coiera[14] identified that communication during handover is consistently inadequate. Knowledge of clinical handover policy is essential in following established structure during communication.

Advanced Practice Nursing

The advanced practice nurse as practitioner, researcher, and educator is responsible for collaborating with both the anesthesia department and the ICU to develop policies and monitor outcomes of IHT.[15] At the project site, the nurse anesthetist directs the process of IHT from the TICU to surgery. Advocating for patient safety and improving the quality of IHT, the advanced practice nurse identifies strengths and weaknesses of the current system. Preventing errors in patient care by assessing knowledge of policy and evaluating the links between practice patterns and policy issues addresses gaps in care that affect patient safety. Analysis of implementation of practice guidelines across the continuum of care for patients requiring IHT is part of the advanced practice nurse role as educator and change advocate.

SYNTHESIS OF BODY OF EVIDENCE RELATED TO THE PROBLEM

IHT of critically ill patients from the ICU for diagnostic tests and procedures is a necessary component of patient care but is associated with adverse events. The reported rates of adverse events range from 5.9% to almost 70.0%[13] and are categorized as mishaps related to patient care (systems based) or physiologic deterioration (patient based). Patient care or systems-based events include equipment and staff issues, such as monitor failure, breathing circuit or airway failure, depleted oxygen supply, underventilation, overventilation, and loss of intravenous access or monitoring.[16,17] Physiologic deterioration or patient-based events included hypoxemia, hypercapnia, heart rhythm changes, blood pressure instability, hypothermia, and poorly managed pain or agitation. Specific events engaging both patient-based and system-based categories include loss of monitoring parameters (eg, pulse oximetry), loss of airway/extubation, oxygen desaturation, tachycardia, bradycardia, hypertension, hypotension, bleeding, and cardiac arrest.

Strengths of the synthesis of the body of knowledge of IHT include the numerous reports of adverse events and categories of failure modes involving the process itself and the critical nature of the patients being transported. Almost 40 years of event reporting during IHT has provided a broad and consistent collection of adverse events ranging from monitor disconnects to cardiac arrest. Guidelines for IHT are well defined and uniform and consistently involve preplanning, adequate and experienced staff, acceptable equipment, continuation of the level of monitoring in the ICU, and communication.[2–5,18] Patient risk factors are well defined and include physiologic instability, mechanical ventilation, and long transports. Recommendations for improving patient safety during IHT consistently include equipment management, team composition, and enhanced communication through education and training.[4,16] Weaknesses of the available evidence include the effect of critical illness on adverse events and outcomes, consistency of adverse event reporting, and the degree to which education and training impacts adverse events and outcomes during IHT. Complicating the assessment of IHT as a safety issue is the confounding effect of patient selection, as these patients typically represent a sicker population. Several reports demonstrate that adverse events may have occurred in these patients whether transported or not.[19–21] Furthermore, definitions of adverse events have been inconsistent, with some studies defining adverse events differently than others. Study populations have been specialty groups, such as cardiac patients or trauma patients. Among these populations, there is a predisposition to a higher incidence of dysrhythmias or desaturation. The benefit of education is not established, and there are no outcome studies demonstrating the effect of standardized communication on decreasing the risk of IHT.[22] The destination and/or origin of IHT may affect adverse events and outcome, as transport to the operating room may be less associated with adverse events than transport from the operating room. These weaknesses must be considered with any review.

Other than the development and description of dedicated IHT teams, there are no reports of interventions that have proven successful in minimizing risks of IHT.[13,23] Despite identification of risks of IHT and guidelines in place since 1999, no other interventions or viable solutions have been identified for the 5.9% to 70.0% incidence of adverse events during IHT. Limitations of reports range from a lack of generalizability (IHT to radiology, from neurology care, from the emergency department) to overreporting of trivial events as adverse (eg, tangled lines, electrocardiogram [ECG] disconnect). There is little research to support the scope of problems encountered during IHT, as the definition of terms, classification of reporting, and varying qualifications of the transport team have been very diverse. Although handover issues are well described, no clear cause or solution has been identified.[22] Assessment of IHT as a safety behavior would begin with eliciting knowledge of the organization's safety policies and training.

CONCEPTS AND DEFINITIONS

IHT is associated with adverse events and is a patient safety issue. Patient safety is an outcome associated with patient care (safety behavior) resulting from a safety culture established by the provider (nurse) and the organization (hospital) as described by Cooper's Reciprocal Safety Culture Model (RSCM).[24] Guidelines for IHT exist to improve patient safety and involve 5 elements as described by Ott and colleagues.[7] Despite guidelines and policies for effective IHT and clinical handover, barriers exist and may involve knowledge of these guidelines, policies, and procedures. Assessment of nursing knowledge of IHT and clinical handover policies may help to identify knowledge deficits of IHT providers that may affect patient safety during IHT. The following are concepts and definitions used during this project:

- IHT is the transportation of patients within a hospital for the purpose of undergoing diagnostic or therapeutic procedures (www.AHRQ.gov). Continuity of care and safe IHT is based on guidelines including preplanning, personnel, equipment, monitoring, and documentation. Core elements or procedures involved in IHT include team composition, patient considerations, handovers, equipment, communication, and minimization of risk.[16]
- *Preplanning* is the "coordination and communication between the sending and the receiving units."[7(p50)]
- *Personnel* is staffing required for IHT, and composition varies depending on whether patients are mechanically ventilated or unstable.[7]
- *Equipment* refers to monitors, ventilators, drug infusions, airway devices, and other physical apparatus used to maintain the same level of care during IHT as in the ICU.[7]
- *Monitoring* refers to "the maintenance of the same level of physiologic monitoring as in the ICU, such as blood pressure, pulse oximetry, cardiac monitoring and arterial lines."[7(p50)]
- *Communication* refers to the exchange of timely and accurate information at transitions of care between providers to optimize safety and continuity of patient care and includes information about patient status and patient-specific considerations.[7(p53)]
- *Clinical handover* is defined as "the transfer of information (along with authority and responsibility) during transitions and care across a continuum; to include an opportunity to ask questions, clarify and confirm" (www.AHRQ.gov).
- *Adverse events* are defined as equipment malfunction, patient physiologic decline of blood pressure, heart rate or oxygen saturation compared with before transport, or any critical situation requiring urgent therapeutic intervention during IHT.[5]
- *Patient safety* is the avoidance, prevention, and amelioration of adverse outcomes or injuries stemming from the process of health care.[11]

- *Knowledge* is defined as familiarity with something, which includes facts, information, description, or skills acquired through education or experience. It can refer to theoretic or practical understanding of a subject (www.merriam-webster.com).

APPLICATION OF THEORETIC FRAMEWORK

In this project, the RSCM[24] provided structure for examining the behaviors and processes of IHT. Cooper's model (**Fig. 1**, Cooper's RSCM) posits patient safety is multi-factorial and maintenance of a safety culture depends on provider, organization, and role of the provider within the organization. Safety is determined by 3 elements: safety management (regulated by the organization), safety climate (regulated by the individual provider), and safety behavior (regulated by the role of the individual provider within the organization). Safety management is established by identifying standard operating procedures or policies (eg, IHT and clinical handover policies). Safety climate is established by verifying knowledge and competence of IHT and clinical handover policies and procedures. Safety behavior is established by observation or self-reporting of independent providers following specific IHT guidelines, including preplanning, use of qualified personnel, vigilant physiologic monitoring, handover with effective communication, and availability of appropriate equipment.

Elements of IHT may be applied to Cooper's model as they relate to the organization, provider, and role of provider within the organization. Preplanning, as a safety behavior before IHT, depends on the organization having a policy dictating coordination and communication as well as the provider having knowledge of the policy. Effective clinical handover as a safety behavior may not occur without understanding effective handover strategies and standardized structure. Recognition of IHT risk requires anticipatory guidance and communication between providers. Effective

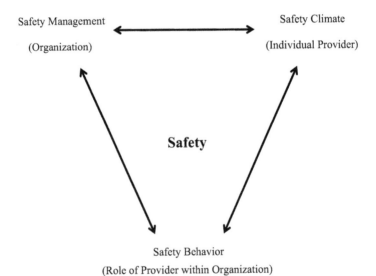

Fig. 1. Cooper's RSCM. Safety is determined by safety management (regulated by the organization), safety climate (regulated by the individual provider), and safety behavior (regulated by the role of the provider within the organization). (*Adapted from* Cooper M. Toward a model of safety culture. Saf Sci 2000;36:120; with permission.)

management of personnel is contingent on the organization having policies in place regarding situational team composition and the provider having knowledge of the content of these policies. Assembling proper equipment and medications for IHT depends on providers knowing their role based on policies generated by the organization. The anesthesia provider must have training to use medications for sedation and hemodynamic management as well as IHT equipment, including airway devices. Maintaining adequate monitoring during IHT requires knowledge of criteria for instability based on policy as well as provider knowledge of appropriate monitoring techniques. Documentation and clinical handover depend on policies being in place and the providers' familiarity with the content and structure of SBAR. In summary, overall execution of the 5 core IHT elements and safety behavior may actually be a composite of safety climate determined by the health care provider and safety management in place by the organization and knowledge of interrelated elements of IHT (**Fig. 2**, Cooper's RSCM and the project).

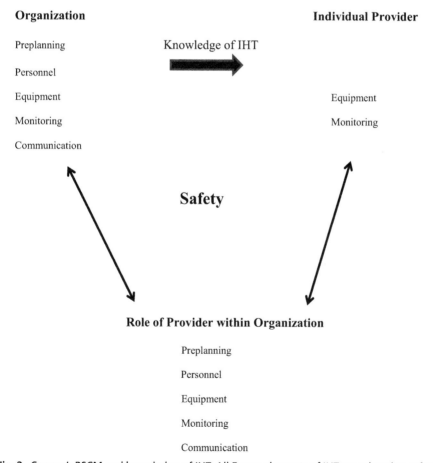

Fig. 2. Cooper's RSCM and knowledge of IHT. All 5 core elements of IHT are related to safety management by the organization, whereas some equipment and monitoring knowledge are elements of the individual provider's role in ICU and surgery. (*From* Cooper M. Toward a model of safety culture. Saf Sci 2000;36:120; with permission.)

METHODOLOGY
Project Design

The purpose of this project was to assess IHT knowledge of nurses, nurse anesthetists, and student nurse anesthetists (SRNAs) working in the trauma subspecialty at the project hospital. The TICU was selected based on the frequency of IHT (397 IHT in a 6-month period). This project was a nonexperimental cross-sectional design using a survey to gather data. The hospital's Institutional Review Board approved the project before survey distribution. The sampling frame included all nurses currently working in the TICU, all nurse anesthetists working within the trauma subspecialty, and all SNRAs on rotation with the trauma service. A convenience sample of participants was used composed of TICU nurses, nurse anesthetists, and student nurse anesthetists. Recruitment of potential subjects was accomplished with the aid of the TICU educator, anesthesia department educator, and the dean of the nurse anesthesia school.

The method used to send and return surveys was Web based and used the REDCap survey system and project hospital's e-mail structure. Steps in the process of data collection were (1) distribution of an e-mail with the survey as a link within an e-mail requesting participation and assuring confidentiality; (2) a reminder in the form of an e-mail 1 week after the survey was generated to the nonrespondents encouraging them to respond; (3) final e-mail with notification of completion of the survey 11 days after the original distribution.

Data Collection

The 5 elements of IHT guided the survey development. Knowledge of IHT and clinical handover policy was assessed through questions regarding preplanning (coordination, communication), personnel (roles of providers, team composition), equipment and medication requirements (level of care, equipment and medication requirements), and communication (clinical handover policy including opportunity for questions, uninterrupted communication, anticipatory guidance, and the use of SBAR). The survey was developed using 5 fields for the components of IHT along with a demographics section. Multiple-choice responses were used with one answer allowed for assessing core elements. Multiple selections were allowed for IHT and handover training so that subjects would have the opportunity to describe their answers more fully. The survey consisted of 10 multiple-choice items representing the 5 core elements, with 2 items covering each element (**Fig. 3**, IHT survey). These 10 items were scored on multiple selections with one response allowed and were all closed ended.

Face validity was sought through a pilot survey and subsequent e-mail response of 10 nurse anesthetists and 10 ICU nurses not working on the trauma service. The survey took approximately 10 minutes to complete and included 16 questions. Survey questions were modified based on feedback from participants and included rewording of 2 questions. Content validity was sought earlier in the process of development through a 3-step process.[25] The full content domain of IHT was identified through dialogues with the project committee; IHT items were generated from all 5 elements; and the instrument was developed by assimilating the items into a useable form as a survey.

Data Analysis of Results

On completion of data collection, statistical analysis was performed using SPSS to determine and measure frequencies and central tendencies. Chi-square tests for independence were used to compare results of the survey. Data gathered included

Confidential

Intrahospital Transport Assessment

Please complete the survey below.

Thank you!

1) Who determines whether a trauma ICU patient is transported to the holding room or directly to the operating room for surgery?

    ☐ Primary ICU nurse caring for patient
    ☐ Nurse anesthetist providing the anesthetic
    ☐ Attending anesthesiologist
    ☐ Primary surgeon

2) What preplanning should occur before a mechanically ventilated patient is transported from the trauma ICU to surgery?

    ☐ Operating room circulating nurse calls the ICU clerk and schedules case
    ☐ Anesthesiologist and surgeon plan transport
    ☐ Transport times are coordinated by the nurse anesthetist and ICU nurse
    ☐ Respiratory therapy coordinates transport with the nurse anesthetist

3) Stable trauma ICU patients scheduled for surgery

    ☐ may be transported to the holding room if mechanically ventilated by a respiratory therapist without an anesthesia provider
    ☐ are evaluated by an anesthesiologist to determine suitability for transport to holding room or direct to the operating room
    ☐ are transported to holding room unless directed by the surgeon
    ☐ never require an anesthesia provider unless mechanically ventilated

4) Transportation of the mechanically ventilated patient from the trauma ICU to surgery

    ☐ always requires at least three personnel
    ☐ may require an ICU nurse if there are not enough anesthesia department staff
    ☐ never requires more than three providers regardless of the patient's condition
    ☐ does not require airway equipment such as a mask if already intubated

5) Medication, monitors and other equipment for transport of the trauma ICU patient to surgery

    ☐ are always provided by the ICU nurse
    ☐ are always provided by anesthesia if being transported directly to the operating room
    ☐ are supplied by the ICU nurse if assisting with the transport
    ☐ are only necessary if the patient is unstable or is mechanically ventilated

6) You are transporting a mechanically ventilated trauma ICU patient to surgery (10 minute transport). How much oxygen should be available in the oxygen transport tank?

    ☐ 20 minutes (tank will be exchanged in surgery)
    ☐ 30 minutes (10 minute reserve)
    ☐ 40 minutes
    ☐ Full tank

7) Which of the following monitors is necessary for transporting mechanically ventilated trauma ICU patients directly to the operating room?

    ☐ Transport monitor with ECG and SpO$_2$ capabilities, blood pressure if there is already an arterial line
    ☐ Transport monitor with ECG, SpO$_2$ and noninvasive blood pressure capability
    ☐ Transport monitor with defibrillator if mechanically ventilated
    ☐ Transport monitor with either ECG or pulse oximeter

Fig. 3. IHT survey. SpO$_2$, blood oxygen saturation. Available at: http://www.project. redcap.org.

demographic information of participating providers, knowledge of core elements of IHT and clinical handover procedures specified in policies, and description of completed education and training. Comparison of providers included years of experience in the current role at the hospital and provider type (ICU nurse, nurse anesthetist, or student nurse anesthetist), along with IHT experience (number of transports). Primary outcomes measured were nurse knowledge of policies including the 5 core elements of IHT, whereas secondary outcomes included provider comparisons and survey performance based on experience and training.

8) Which of the following scenarios may not require an anesthesia provider for transport from the trauma ICU to surgery?

- ☐ Infusion of normal saline at 500 mL/hour
- ☐ Norepinephrine infusion 2 mcg/minute for last 48 hours
- ☐ Neck or facial injury with potential airway issue
- ☐ PO_2 100 mm Hg on 50% face mask
- ☐ The surgeon considers the patient to be unstable

9) Which of the following is a required component of the clinical handover prior to transporting a trauma ICU patient to surgery?

- ☐ Information is prepared in advance by the trauma ICU nurse if not personally handing over the patient
- ☐ Verbal or text report of access, continuous infusions and significant lab values
- ☐ Review of the electronic preop by the anesthesia provider along with any updates from the trauma ICU nurse
- ☐ The trauma ICU nurse offers anticipatory guidance to the nurse anesthetist

10) SBAR is an acronym that refers to

- ☐ Subjective information, background of current illness, analysis of clinical data and review of patient history
- ☐ A checklist of tasks to be performed prior to transition of care
- ☐ A method for the exchange of information during transitions of care
- ☐ Verbal report provided when the patient is mechanically ventilated

11) How many times have you transported a patient being mechanically ventilated directly from the trauma ICU to surgery?

- ☐ Less than five
- ☐ 5-10
- ☐ 10-20
- ☐ >20

12) Age

- ☐ < 25 years old
- ☐ 25-30 years old
- ☐ 30-40 years old
- ☐ 40-50 years old
- ☐ > 50 years old

13) Current Provider Role

- ☐ ICU nurse
- ☐ Nurse anesthetist
- ☐ Student nurse anesthetist

14) How long have you been practicing in your current role at Vanderbilt University Medical Center?

- ☐ Less than one year
- ☐ Less than 2 years
- ☐ Less than 3 years
- ☐ More than 3 years

15) What training have you received for intrahospital transport?

- ☐ Checklist or handout
- ☐ Vandysafe or web inservice
- ☐ Part of orientation
- ☐ Other
- ☐ None

16) What training have you received for clinical handover?

- ☐ Checklist or handout
- ☐ Vandysafe or web inservice
- ☐ Part of orientation
- ☐ Other
- ☐ None

Fig. 3. (*continued*)

After obtaining approval from the hospital's Institutional Review Board, 80 TICU nurses, 64 student nurse anesthetists, and 58 nurse anesthetists working in the trauma service were asked to participate. Of these 202 potential subjects, 119 (59%) completed the survey (**Table 1**, demographics). Descriptive statistical frequencies and percentages were used to analyze the survey items for knowledge of IHT. The survey items were grouped according to the core element each item was intended to measure. Responses were organized according to provider type and combined for overall response rates to assess for knowledge of IHT and compared using chi-square test for independence (**Table 2**, responses to survey questions).

Table 1 Demographics		
Surveys Distributed	**Surveys Returned**	**Percentage (%)**
202	119	59
Provider role	Frequency	Percent
TICU nurse	40	34
CRNA	42	35
SRNA	37	31
Experience with IHT	Frequency	Percent
<5 transports	25	21
5–10 transports	23	19
10–20 transports	12	10
>20 transports	59	50
Years in current role		
Less than 1 y	26	22
Less than 2 y	23	18
Less than 3 y	22	18
More than 3 y	49	41

RESULTS

In assessing nurse knowledge of IHT, the 5 core elements were evaluated using 10 survey items. The subjects' answers were analyzed for frequencies and correct response. Overall performance on the assessment was calculated along with selection to determine knowledge and standardization between providers and provider groups. For each item, a correct answer based on the hospital's policy was either selected or not selected and a correct answer percentage generated for the entire sample as well as provider groups. In analyzing for failure modes, such as inadequate planning, insufficient team composition, equipment failure, level of monitoring, and communication errors, specific selection frequencies were evaluated (**Table 2**, responses to survey questions). The 5 core elements were used to guide this project as well as the survey questions. The results from the subjects' responses are discussed in relation to the core element it represents.

Core Element 1: Preplanning

Preplanning for IHT includes determination of who is transported directly to surgery and communication between the TICU nurse and anesthesia. Coordination and communication between the sending and receiving units is essential to transfer information about patient status, specific needs, and personnel requirements. Fifty percent of all providers correctly selected the anesthesiologist as making the determination of who is transported direct to surgery by IHT, whereas 35% incorrectly selected the surgeon (including 55% of the nurse anesthetists). Seventy-four percent correctly identified that preplanning occurs between the TICU nurse and nurse anesthetist, with 19% selecting the surgeon and anesthesiologist (26% of the nurse anesthetists).

Core Element 2: Personnel

Personnel requirements and provider roles include who transports and how many staff are required. Critically ill patients require an evaluation by an anesthesiologist

Table 2
Responses to survey questions

IHT Core Element	TICU Nurse n = 40	CRNA n = 42	SRNA n = 37	Overall n = 119
Planning 1: Who designates patients as direct to surgery by IHT?				
Correct answer	43%	31%	81%	50%
A. Primary ICU nurse	2	6	2	10 (8%)
B. CRNA	6	0	1	7 (6%)
C. Anesthesiologist	**17**	**13**	**30[a]**	**60 (50%)**
D. Surgeon	15	23	4	42 (35%)
Planning 2: Who is involved in preplanning before IHT?				
Correct answer	83%	74%	65%	74%
A. Circulator	2	0	0	2 (2%)
B. Surgeon and anesthesiologist	5	11	7	23 (19%)
C. CRNA and TICU nurse	**33[a]**	**31**	**24**	**88 (74%)**
D. CRNA and respiratory therapist	0	0	6	6 (5%)
Personnel 1: Stable TICU patients are transported to surgery				
Correct answer	48%	52%	92%	63%
A. Respiratory therapy to holding without anesthesia if stable	2	1	0	3 (3%)
B. Evaluated by anesthesiologist before transport for IHT or holding	**19**	**22**	**34[a]**	**75 (63%)**
C. Transported to holding unless directed by surgeon	5	5	1	11 (9%)
D. Never require anesthesia unless mechanically ventilated	14	14	2	30 (25%)
Personnel 2: What personnel are required for transportation of mechanically ventilated patients to surgery?				
Correct answer	45%	83%	92%	73%
A. Always requires at least 3 staff	**18**	**35**	**34[a]**	**87 (73%)**
B. Requires TICU nurse if not enough anesthesia staff	22	7	3	32 (27%)
C. Never requires more than 3 staff	0	0	0	0 (0%)

D. Does not require airway equipment if already intubated	0	0	0	0 (0%)
Equipment 1: What equipment considerations exist for IHT?				
Correct answer	93%	100%	100%	98%
A. Equipment is always provided by TICU nurse	1	0	0	1 (1%)
B. Equipment is always provided by anesthesia if going to OR	37	42	37	116 (98%)
C. Equipment is supplied by TICU nurse if assisting with IHT	2	0	0	2 (2%)
D. Equipment is only necessary if unstable or if mechanically ventilated	0	0	0	0 (0%)
Equipment 2: How much oxygen is required for IHT?				
Correct answer	3%	7%	3%	4%
A. 20 min	0	0	0	0 (0%)
B. 30 min	0	2	2	4 (3%)
C. 40 min	1	3	1	5 (4%)
D. Full tank	39	37	34	110 (92%)
Monitoring 1: What monitoring is required for IHT of mechanically ventilated patients?				
Correct answer	53%	62%	70%	65%
A. Transport monitor with ECG, pulse oximeter, BP if preexisting arterial line present	18	16	11	45 (38%)
B. Transport monitor with ECG, oxygen saturation, noninvasive BP capability	21	26	26	73 (61%)
C. Transport monitor with defibrillator if mechanically ventilated	1	0	0	1 (1%)
D. Attending anesthesiologist if on any dose of vasopressin	0	0	0	0 (0%)
Monitoring 2: Which scenario does not require anesthesia for IHT?				
Correct answer	43%	33%	30%	35%
A. Infusion of normal saline at 500 mL/h	16	17	22	55 (46%)
B. Norepinephrine infusion @ 2 mcg/min for 48 h	6	10	3	19 (16%)
C. Neck or facial injury with potential airway issue	0	0	0	0 (0%)
D. Po_2 100 mm Hg on 50% face tent	17	14	11	42 (35%)
E. The surgeon considers patients unstable	1	0	1	2 (2%)

(continued on next page)

Table 2
(continued)

IHT Core Element	TICU Nurse $n = 40$	CRNA $n = 42$	SRNA $n = 37$	Overall $n = 119$
Communication 1: What is a required component of clinical handover for IHT?				
Correct answer	3%	8%	0%	4%
A. Information prepared by ICU nurse if checklist used by unit	8	1	3	12 (10%)
B. Verbal or text report of access, laboratory values, infusions	10	12	2	24 (20%)
C. Anesthesia reviews EMR and asks for any missing information	21	26	32	79 (66%)
D. The ICU nurse offers anticipatory guidance	1	3[a]	0	4 (3%)
Communication 2: What does the acronym SBAR represent?				
Correct answer	70%	45%	68%	62%
A. Subjective information, background of illness, analysis of data, review of history	11	23	12	46 (39%)
B. Checklist of tasks before IHT	0	0	0	0 (0%)
C. Method of exchange of information before transitions of care	28	19	25	72 (61%)
D. Verbal report for when patients are mechanically ventilated	1	0	0	1 (1%)

Note: Correct answer in boldface.

Abbreviations: BP, blood pressure; CRNA, certified registered nurse anesthetist; EMR, electronic medical record; OR, operating room.

[a] $P<.01$ compared with other groups.

and a minimum of 3 staff for transport. An anesthesia provider is required for mechanically ventilated and unstable patients along with the primary ICU nurse. Sixty-three percent of all providers recognized that an anesthesiologist must evaluate patients before transport if mechanically ventilated, whereas 25% did not know unstable patients require anesthesia personnel for transport (33% of nurse anesthetists). Seventy-three percent recognized that 3 providers are required, whereas 27% did not know the primary nurse is to accompany patients during transport (55% of the TICU nurses).

Core Element 3: Equipment

Equipment is always the responsibility of anesthesia personnel during IHT, whereas oxygen supply is a responsibility shared by the TICU nurse and nurse anesthetist. Equipment must be confirmed to be in working order, and all nurses must be proficient in its use. Ninety-eight percent of all providers knew that anesthesia personnel are responsible for the equipment for IHT. Four percent knew that policy dictates a 40-minute supply of oxygen is required for IHT. Ninety-two percent of all providers selected full tank as the requirement for IHT instead of a 40-minute supply. A full tank holds approximately 660 L of oxygen, whereas only 320 L is required.

Core Element 4: Monitoring

Monitoring requirements stipulate that patients being transported must have their blood pressure monitored at the same frequency as it was monitored in the ICU. Sixty-one percent of all providers selected blood pressure monitoring as being a requirement for IHT. Thirty-eight percent only monitor blood pressure if an invasive arterial blood pressure is available. Unstable patients based on criteria established by policy require anesthesia personnel for IHT. Forty-four percent of respondents correctly selected adequate oxygenation using a face tent delivery system as not requiring anesthesia personnel. Forty-six percent selected a patient being fluid resuscitated (infusion of normal saline at 500 mL/h) as being stable for transport without anesthesia personnel.

Core Element 5: Communication

Communication and handover requires interactive, structured 2-way communication with anticipatory guidance. Without communication of patient information and anticipatory guidance, inappropriate interventions or errors may occur. Three percent of all providers selected anticipatory guidance as a component of clinical handover, whereas the majority (66%) selected a review of the medical record and request for any missing information. Sixty-one percent of all respondents recognized SBAR as a method of communication before transitions of care, whereas the other 39% selected an option that contained words used in conversation beginning with SBAR.

In analyzing all 5 core elements, the correct response rate for all nurses and provider groups averaged 53%. TICU nurses and nurse anesthetists scored 80% or higher in 2 of the 10 elements. SNRAs scored 80% or higher in 4 of the 10 elements. Average scores for the TICU nurses, nurse anesthetists, and SNRAs were 48%, 59%, and 60%, respectively.

Significant differences in responses to survey questions were found between provider groups in core elements of IHT. SNRAs were more likely than TICU nurses or nurse anesthetists to know who determines cases in which a patient is taken direct to surgery. A chi-square test of independence was performed to examine the relationship between provider type and knowledge of who determines that a patient is taken direct to surgery. The relation between these variables was significant,

χ^2 (6, N = 119) = 32.84, $P<.01$. The TICU nurse is more likely than the SRNA or nurse anesthetist to know who is to communicate immediately before IHT to plan the transport. A chi-square test of independence was performed to examine the relationship between provider type and knowledge of which providers should plan the IHT. The relation between these variables was significant, χ^2 (6, N = 119) = 20.05, $P<.01$.

SRNAs were more likely than TICU nurses or nurse anesthetists to know what mechanism is involved in transporting mechanically ventilated patients to surgery. Ninety-two percent of all SRNAs correctly selected evaluation of an anesthesiologist is required for all IHT to surgery regardless of whether ventilated, compared with 52% of nurse anesthetists and 48% of TICU nurses. A chi-square test of independence was performed to examine the relationship between provider type and knowledge of when anesthesia transports patients directly to the operating room. The relation between these variables was significant, χ^2 (6, N = 119) = 17.73, $P<.01$. Ninety-two percent of all SRNAs correctly selected 3 staff requirements for IHT, compared with 83% of all nurse anesthetists and 45% of all TICU nurses. A chi-square test of independence was performed to examine the relationship between provider type and knowledge of staffing requirements for IHT. The relation between these variables was significant, χ^2 (2, N = 119) = 24.95, $P<.01$.

Nurse anesthetists were more likely than TICU nurses or SRNAs to know what components of clinical handover are mandated by policy. A chi-square test of independence was performed to examine the relationship between provider type and knowledge of clinical handover components. The relation between these variables was significant, χ^2 (6, N = 119) = 19.11, $P<.01$. Although statistically significant, only 7% of nurse anesthetists correctly selected anticipatory guidance as a component.

No significant differences in responses to survey questions were found among providers with different levels of IHT experience. Of the respondents, 8 nurse anesthetists, 5 TICU nurses, and 1 SNRA had no IHT training. No significant differences existed in results for providers with IHT training (checklists, Web-based in-service, or orientation) and those with no IHT training or between different modalities of training (Web based, orientation, or other training).

DISCUSSION OF PROJECT RESULTS
Relationship of Project Results to Theoretic Framework

The purpose of this survey was to assess nurse knowledge of IHT composed of 5 core elements established through policy. The survey measured 2 items of each core element of IHT and assessed overall performance, the effect of different provider groups, the effect of experience level, and the effect of IHT training. Each element is a component of Cooper's RSCM, and knowledge of these elements is essential in promoting safety behavior within a safety culture. Consistent with the theoretic framework, equipment and monitoring knowledge is similar in all 3 provider groups. Equipment refers to monitors, ventilators, and other physical apparatus used during IHT; equipment knowledge is similar among all provider groups working in the trauma service. Knowledge of monitoring considerations is similar such that this element is related more to the individual provider than to the organization. Knowledge of these elements does not vary significantly between providers as demonstrated by the survey and analysis. The analysis of survey results also demonstrates differences in 3 core elements of IHT among the provider groups: preplanning, personnel requirements, and communication. Knowledge of these 3 elements and policies differ significantly among providers, whereas no differences exist because of experience with IHT or training.

Impact of Results on Practice

The impact of the results of this study on the practice of IHT is related to the importance of knowledge of policy. This study highlighted serious knowledge deficits, which have the potential to threaten patient safety and reduce the effectiveness of IHT. Through analyzing the results in a clinical context, failure modes may be related to the knowledge of policy of the provider primarily responsible for a particular element of IHT. Preplanning is initiated by the nurse anesthetist or SNRA before IHT, with the anesthesiologist determining whether patients are transported direct to surgery. The nurse anesthetist incorrectly selected the person determining the method of transport 69% of the time. Personnel requirements and IHT team composition are managed by all 3 providers and include 3 staff members, including the TICU nurse. Fifty-five percent of TICU nurses did not know the primary ICU nurse is to assist in transporting patients. Sixty-seven percent of the nurse anesthetists did not know the anesthesia provider transports unstable patients from the ICU to surgery regardless of airway status. The ICU nurse is responsible for offering anticipatory guidance to the anesthesia provider, but only one TICU nurse selected this answer (2.5%). Patient safety may be compromised, as individual providers responsible for safety behaviors are not familiar with policy.

Knowledge of policy is inconsistent among provider groups, and the results of this survey indicate a need for knowledge translation. Although 106 of 119 responders indicated they had received IHT training, differences existed between provider groups. IHT training must be incongruent among providers and may affect knowledge and practice patterns. A significant finding in this survey is the relationship of structured training and orientation to IHT knowledge. The least experienced provider (SRNAs) scored higher than the hospital's employees (TICU nurses and nurse anesthetists) on 4 of the 10 items and possessed the highest average score. Although certified registered nurse anesthetists (CRNAs) and TICU nurses received orientation to IHT, SRNAs as a group received specific training for clinical handover, SBAR, and IHT, which included PowerPoint (Microsoft Corporation, Redmond, WA) presentations, a Web-based in-service, and a written examination including IHT. In addition, the SRNAs were required to demonstrate proper SBAR use and participate in 2 IHT transports before completing orientation. Participation in a similar enhanced training course for all providers may improve knowledge of IHT policy.

Overall Strengths and Weaknesses of Project

Strengths of this project include the use of IHT and clinical handover policies to guide the survey development. IHT core elements and Cooper's RSCM were to construct the 10 items used to assess nurse knowledge. Use of the IHT policy provides a universal format for all 3 provider groups as the policy applies to all providers. In addition, survey participants included only TICU nurses, nurse anesthetists, and SNRAs in the trauma service. In this manner, all IHT members were represented and provider differences were captured. Analysis of the participants' responses provides an overall assessment of nurse knowledge of the IHT policy.

The survey was based on objective data contained within the actual policy itself, and the response format included only one correct answer. Multiple-choice questions were used, a format common to all groups for licensure, certification, and Web-based in-services. Two experts in the development of assessment tools reviewed the survey before use for reliability, clarity, grammar errors, wording, test format, and relevance to the policies. Face validity was established before using the survey for the project through a pilot survey of a similar group of specialized ICU nurses and nurse anesthetists.

The survey process included an e-mail notifying the participant of the survey as a link in the thread of the e-mail and encouraged participation without disclosing its components. The researcher was named, and the purpose of the survey identified as being used to develop a quality-improvement project involving IHT. No mention was made of the IHT or clinical handover policies or that the survey was actually a knowledge assessment. The second notification via e-mail again contained wording about development of a quality-improvement project and encouraging participation of invitees. The final notification thanked everyone for their participation and encouraged those who had not participated to take the survey on its last day. More than 58% of invitees responded from 3 separate provider groups, with representation of all provider groups.

Weaknesses of the project include the use of an untested survey. Reliability has not been established for the survey; because of this, the degree to which the survey captures true knowledge of IHT is unknown. Provider subcultures and roles may also affect decision making and knowledge. Pidgeon and O'Leary[26] recognized organizational differentiation into subcultures, which can influence perceptions of guidelines and skew knowledge. In this manner, TICU nurses may interpret IHT and clinical handover policies differently than interpretation of the nurse anesthetists. The survey was offered in an uncontrolled environment in which the participant potentially had access to the policies and could verify information while actually taking the survey. In addition there was no time limit for the survey, and there may have been lower scores in a controlled environment without warning as to content or purpose. Implications for poor performance or not being a safe practitioner may have affected the results and participation. The Rosenthal effect may have potentially affected results, but the surveyor had minimal interaction with the participants.

Future Implications for Practice

Surveys have been used previously to assess for knowledge of nursing practice, including blood transfusion, nutrition, and chest drain care.[27–29] These surveys measured knowledge of best practice based on existing literature but not specific policy or guidelines. Assessment of nursing knowledge based on literature for evidence-based practice may not be relevant because of barriers to research utilization, such as resources, time, and comprehension.[30]

In an era of evidence-based practice and accountability, safety policies are developed to establish comprehensive guidelines. As clinical decision making is based more on best practice and policy, knowledge of policies is essential. The first step involved in improving the quality of patient care is investigating and documenting the current state of knowledge of the providers. Assessment of policy knowledge and understanding may provide a vehicle for raising staff awareness, identifying strengths and areas for improvement, and to conduct internal and external comparisons between provider groups. Findings may then be used to plan and implement educational programs based on the nurses' specific needs. Furthermore the findings may be used to revise, upgrade, and strengthen policy and guidelines.

REFERENCES

1. Voigt L, Pastores S, Raoof N, et al. Intra-hospital transport of critically ill patients: Outcomes, timing and patterns. J Intensive Care Med 2009;24:108–15.
2. Waydhas C. Intrahospital transport of critically ill patients. Crit Care 1999;3:83–9. Available at: http//ccforum.com.
3. Warren J, Fromm R, Orr R, et al. Guidelines for the inter-and intrahospital transport of critically ill patients. Crit Care Med 2004;32:256–62.

4. Papson JP, Russell KL, Taylor D. Unexpected events during the intrahospital transport of patients. Acad Emerg Med 2007;14:574–7.
5. Fanara B, Manzon C, Barbot O, et al. Recommendations for the intra-hospital transport of critically ill patients. Crit Care 2010;14(R87):1–10.
6. Borowitz SM, Waggoner-Fountain LA, Bass EJ, et al. Adequacy of information transferred at resident sign-out (in-hospital handover of care): a prospective survey. Qual Saf Health Care 2006;17:6–10.
7. Ott L, Hoffman L, Hravnak M. Intrahospital transport to the radiology department: risk for adverse events, nursing surveillance, utilization of a MET, and practice implications. J Radiol Nurs 2011;30:49–54.
8. Beckman U, Gillies D, Berenholtz S, et al. Incidents relating to the intra-hospital transport of critically ill patients: an analysis of the reports submitted to the Australian Incident Monitoring Study in Intensive Care. Intensive Care Med 2004;30:1579–85.
9. Agency for Healthcare Research and Quality. Making healthcare safer: a critical analysis of patient safety practices. 2001. Available at: http://archive.ahrq.gov/clinic/ptsafety/pdf/ptsafety.pdf. Accessed January 13, 2013.
10. American Association of Critical Care Nurses. Guidelines for the transfer of critically ill patients. Am J Crit Care 1993;2:189–95.
11. Institute of Medicine. To err is human: building a safer health system. Washington, DC: National Academy Press; 2000.
12. Institute of Medicine. Crossing the quality chasm: a new health system for the 21st century. Washington, DC: National Academy Press; 2001.
13. McLenon M. Use of a specialized transport team for intrahospital transport of critically ill patients. Dimens Crit Care Nurs 2004;23:225–9.
14. Ong M, Coiera E. A systematic review of failures in handoff communication during intrahospital transfers. Joint Comm J Qual Patient Saf 2011;37:274–84.
15. Caruana M, Culp K. Intrahospital transport of the critically ill adult: a research review and implications. Dimens Crit Care Nurs 1998;17:146–56.
16. Day D. Keeping patients safe during intrahospital transport. Crit Care Nurse 2010;30(4):18–32.
17. Evans A, Winslow E. Oxygen saturation and hemodynamic response in critically ill, mechanically ventilated adults during intrahospital transport. Am J Crit Care 1995;4:106–11.
18. Society of Critical Care Medicine. Guidelines for the transfer of critically ill patients. Crit Care Med 1993;21:931–7.
19. Hurst J, Davis K, Johnson D, et al. Cost and complications during in-hospital transport of critically ill patients: a prospective cohort study. J Trauma 1992;33: 582–5.
20. Szem J, Hydo L, Fischer S, et al. High-risk transport of critically ill patients: safety and outcome of the necessary "road trip". Crit Care Med 1995;23:1660–6.
21. Taylor J, Chulay J, Hood W, et al. Monitoring high-risk cardiac patients during transportation in hospital. Lancet 1970;296:1205–8.
22. Reisenberg LA, Leitzsch J, Cunningham JM. Nursing handoffs: a systematic review of the literature. Am J Nurs 2010;110(4):24–34.
23. Kue R, Brown P, Ness C, et al. Adverse clinical events during intrahospital transport by a specialized team: a preliminary report. Am J Crit Care 2011;20: 153–61.
24. Cooper M. Towards a model of safety culture. Saf Sci 2000;36:111–36.
25. Lynn MR. Determination and quantification of content validity. Nurse Res 1986;35: 382–5.

26. Pidgeon N, O'Leary M. Man-made disasters: why technology and organizations (sometimes) fail. Saf Sci 2000;34:15–30.

27. Boaz M, Rychani L, Barami K, et al. Nurses and nutrition: a survey of knowledge and attitudes regarding nutrition assessment and care of hospitalized elderly patients. J Contin Educ Nurs 2013;44:1–8.

28. Hijji B, Oweis A, Dabbour R. Measuring knowledge of blood transfusion: a survey of Jordanian nurses. Am Int J Contemp Res 2012;2:77–94.

29. Lehwaldt D, Timmins F. Nurses' knowledge of chest drain care: an exploratory descriptive survey. Nurs Crit Care 2005;10:192–200.

30. Gerrish K, Clayton J. Promoting evidence-based practice: an organizational approach. J Nurs Manag 2004;12:114–23.

Medication Order Entry and Clinical Decision Support: Current Nursing Informatics Issues

Amy C. Gideon, MS, EdD[a],*, David M. DiPersio, PharmD[b]

KEYWORDS

- Technology • Medication order entry systems • Clinical decision support
- Patient safety

KEY POINTS

- The true benefit to nursing with electronic health records is to integrate data from separate sources into a seamless user-friendly application that displays relevant information in a time-sensitive manner, and provides adequate safeguards to reduce potential misadventures. Commercial database and electronic health record applications have the ability to combine massive amounts of information into clinical decision support (CDS) platforms.
- The ideal CDS does not exist; however, local improvements can be made building onto the existing commercial systems to improve quality. The ideal CDS for a local hospital or health system should, as a baseline, take advantage of all of the meaningful use required benefits offered by commercial CDS systems. Meaningful use objectives are expanding beyond key requirements in commercial systems, and the processes used in developing local enhancements to increase the flexibility of commercial CDS are important for success.
- Options and additional resources for commercial CDS systems include prompts for nurses at point of care, alerts, order entry, electronic access to supporting data for each order and alert, patient education, and patient safety. Nurses and advanced practice nurses should have an open line of communication with the information technology department in their facilities and continue with open dialogue to enhance and support medication order entry (MOE) and CDS system development and refinement whether commercially or homegrown systems are used. The nurse is often the last safety defense for the patient in medication administration.

INTRODUCTION

The Health Information Technology for Economic and Clinical Health (HITECH) Act, legislated as part of the American Recovery and Reinvestment Act of 2009,[1] has

Disclosure Statement: The authors have identified no financial or professional affiliations.
[a] Department of Learning Resources, Middle Tennessee School of Anesthesia, 315 Hospital Drive, Madison, TN 37115, USA; [b] Health IT @VUMC, Vanderbilt University Medical Center, 3401 West End Avenue, Nashville, TN 37203, USA
* Corresponding author.
E-mail address: amy@mtsa.edu

greatly increased the acceptance of electronic health record (EHR) technology by providing incentives and punishment standards.[2] It is easy to speculate that none of the early internally designed (homegrown) legacy computer systems designed in the past 30 years to assist with medical clinical decision support (CDS) have been able to support all of the current and future requirements for order entry to achieve the "meaningful use" criteria as defined by the HITECH Act.[3-5] As such, hospitals and clinics have been rushing to commercial EHR systems (vendor systems) that offer an "out-of-the-box" solution to meet the HITECH requirements. It is likely that all future EHR implementations will use these commercial systems that include continuously updated massive databases.[4]

In the rush to meet the requirements for meaningful use, vendor systems have placed more emphasis on achieving the goals for compliance than on working out details that are clinically meaningful.[6] Many CDS goals meaningful to nurses and nursing informatics have been largely overlooked by the HITECH Act.[7] The true benefit to nursing with EHRs is to integrate data from separate sources into a seamless user-friendly application that displays relevant information in a time-sensitive manner, and provides adequate safeguards to reduce potential misadventures. Nurses need to be collaboratively involved in supporting CDS initiative changes that make patient care more effective and efficient.[8] In this brief review, we discuss some of the key current issues and shortfalls of vendor CDS systems as they relate to nursing, as well as proposed potential solutions.

COMMERCIAL CLINICAL DECISION SUPPORT SYSTEM OVERVIEW

Commercial database and EHR vendors have the ability to include massive amounts of information into CDS platforms.[9] Inventories of currently available drugs and medical supplies with updated commercial bar coding based on National Drug Code have the promise to reduce medical errors.[10] However, a significant number of doses prepared in hospital pharmacies are either repackaged, compounded, or made into admixtures by pharmacists and, because these are locally prepared medications, are not included in commercial databases.[11] Checking drug-drug interactions using details from the US Food and Drug Administration (FDA)-approved package labeling or by vendor clinical team review typically produces interruptive alerts in situations in which a documented patient allergy, proposed drug interaction, or dosing alert is triggered. The number and frequency of these alerts, the lack of patient-specific alert severity and consequence, and the interruptive nature have shown to result in *"alert fatigue"* with a corresponding frequency of alert override rates.[12-14]

Alert Fatigue

By nature, commercial database vendors consider the need to include all known alerts to avoid potential litigation.[15] Supporting evidence for alerts in commercial systems is generally provided as a large text document available on demand that includes standard library citations for sources, but does not generally include active links to Internet sources, thus limiting value in a work setting.

Use of tailored or limited warnings has been proposed as a solution by members of a large informatics group and information is available to suggest that such efforts to eliminate alert fatigue may be possible without an increased risk of litigation.[16] Listings of drug interaction warnings that should be noninterruptive, high priority, and essential for patient safety have been proposed.[14,17,18] Although local hospital and health systems have the ability to create free-form, rules-based approaches to modify and enhance these alert methods, attempting to incorporate this information into a commercial database may be difficult and modifications may be overridden by future database updates.[4]

Patient-Specific Clinical Decision Support Pitfalls

CDS systems often provide handouts for patients, which can be useful for discharge planning; however, such handouts from commercial systems may require printing at specific system printers. Drug information discharge sheets in commercial CDS systems are generally available in English; however, other full information for other languages, including Spanish, may not be available. Additionally, information on drugs used in investigational studies is universally missing from commercial CDS systems.[19]

Although information on dosing approved by the FDA prevents ordering an approved dose of a medication outside of a usual dosage range, many drugs do not have approved dosing for commonly encountered situations, such as approved pediatric dosing, or dosing generally accepted as safe and effective, or dosing used in investigational protocols.[20]

OPTIONS AND ADDITIONAL RESOURCES FOR COMMERCIAL CLINICAL DECISION SUPPORT SYSTEMS

The ideal CDS does not exist; however, local improvements can be made building onto the existing commercial systems to improve quality.[13,21] The ideal CDS for a local hospital or health system should, as a baseline, take advantage of all of the meaningful use required benefits offered by commercial CDS systems. This requires that such things as an active medication list, up-to-date problem list of current and active diagnoses and problems, and documented allergies would be imported when a patient is transferred or received by a hospital or health system.[3] Meaningful use objectives are expanding beyond key requirements in commercial systems, and the processes used in developing local enhancements to increase the flexibility of commercial CDS are important for success.

Prompts for Nurses at Point of Care

The need to incorporate appropriate drug-drug, drug-disease, and location-specific alerting into nursing care workflow has been largely overlooked by commercial CDS systems.[22] Human factors principles, or tailoring the computer systems to the work environment, are proposed to recommend appropriate alert design for individual users.[23] Many drug interaction alerts are designed to notify the prescriber of the need to monitor vital signs to ensure patient safety; however, these alerts also should be presented to the nurse at the appropriate time for administration. For example, an alert might be displayed during order entry warning of the need to monitor respiratory rate in a patient with a history of sleep apnea when an order for morphine is ordered. This warning should be displayed to nurses at the time of medication administration.[24] Such a warning could be suppressed for a patient with a *do not resuscitate* order admitted for comfort care in a hospice setting.[25] When a drug is ordered that might cause complications such as confusion, falls, or urinary retention in an elderly patient,[26] the nurse should be reminded at the time of medication administration to monitor and ask the patient if these complications are problematic. When 2 drugs are ordered that might require monitoring and hold criteria (eg, verapamil and metoprolol), which may have additive effects on lowering blood pressure and heart rate,[27] such a warning should be displayed to the nurse during medication administration. Pregnancy alert warnings for drugs that induce labor, such as misoprostol, should not be displayed in a delivery setting,[28] and rubella-containing vaccines, contraindicated in pregnancy, should not give a warning postpartum.[29] Some patients require use of drug combinations that may increase the risk of developing long QT syndrome (LQTS), a change seen on the electrocardiogram (ECG).[30] LQTS is associated with an increased risk of TdP (torsade de pointes), a malignant cardiac rhythm disorder presenting as polymorphic ventricular tachycardia. TdP can self-terminate, but may progress to cardiac arrest. Electrolyte disturbances (hypokalemia, hypomagnesaemia, hypocalcemia) can predispose a patient to LQTS.[31] During order entry, prescribers could be informed of this risk and shown current electrolyte laboratory values. When drug combinations are used that predispose to LQTS, nurses in cardiac telemetry units should be prompted to monitor the QT interval on the ECG, whereas nurses in other patient care settings should be prompted to monitor for patient dizziness or presyncope.[32]

Infusion *smart pumps* can be programmed and display libraries that include safe patient-specific rate limits for allowable drug concentrations. Infusion pump rates can be set with rate limits that would reduce the risk of programming rates considered potentially harmful or insufficient. These limits can be configured as *"soft stops,"* which prompt a user to consider the entered rate, or *"hard stops,"* which could be bypassed only if a reason or comment is added during pump programming.[33] Likewise, dosages for drugs not given by infusion can be set to allow entry of common accepted doses for an individual drug, but also will provide dosing suggestions if these dosage limits are exceeded.[34] Systems should be able to track when each alert notification displays and create a log of user actions to allow retrospective auditing. Alerts deemed excessive or of little clinical value should be changed or eliminated if auditing shows them to be ineffective or lead to alert fatigue.[14,17]

There are advantages and disadvantages for each method of electronically charting medication administration and documenting nursing contact notes.[35] The use of multiple locations for electronic patient access, such as at a secure point-of-care area, on a mobile cart, or in a central location might be considered based on need.[36]

Clinical Decision Support Improvements

Several tools and concepts can be used to locally improve or supplement CDS. Local initiatives should conform to standard terminology to allow electronic exchange (interoperability) of clinical health information. RXNORM is a standard coding system for drugs, Logical Observation Identifiers Names and Codes (LOINC) for laboratory tests,[37] Systemic Nomenclature of Medicine (SNOMED) for clinical terminology,[38] and International Classification of Diseases (ICD) codes[39] for disease states.

Alerts

For example, although a commercial CDS system might present an allergy alert in a patient with penicillin or a codeine allergy, use of a drug that is similar to that drug should give an alert, at least initially, if prescribed. If it is determined that a similar drug is found to be tolerated without undue incident, the system should be able to suppress future false-positive allergy warnings for drugs known to be tolerated. Therefore, it is important to enable trigger-alert drug groups that have a similar characteristic and by individual drugs.[13]

Local CDS systems benefit most if the uses of passive, noninterruptive alerts are used. With passive alerts, the CDS directs the user to the most appropriate practices unobtrusively. The most common use of passive alerts is use of order sets, which not only speed order entry and review, but also ensure that all necessary orders (ie, diet and activity orders) are not omitted.

Order Entry

Incorporation of laboratory, demographic, diagnosis, and genomic information through an automatic interface can improve meaningful and timely suggestions during order entry. Patient-specific genetic variants have been shown to affect drug efficacy or toxicity for a number of drugs.[40] If genomic information is known, such advice might prove useful in guiding individualized drug therapy. Values from common chemistry can be screened and converted by mathematical functions, such as use of age, weight, and serum creatinine to estimate renal function. Laboratory values, vital signs, and trends (eg, increases in creatinine over time) might be incorporated into orders and issue prompts to modify therapy. This information can be incorporated as a prompt during order entry. For example, if a drug is ordered on a child, the set of order suggestions should be limited to appropriate age-based and weight-based options. An adult with reduced renal function would be given a different set of orders, with a desirable default set (eg, dosage form, route, frequencies, dose, and duration) based on the laboratory and diagnosis. Pertinent current laboratory values would be displayed on the same order screen, but would not interrupt the ordering process unless critical. Alerts deemed critical may include severe allergies or protocol violations and could be made interruptive. Use of colors, size, location, and severity can be used to emphasize the importance of the alert. To improve workflow during order entry, the specific alert might suggest discontinuation or modification of the order being entered. Discontinuing or modifying a preexisting order or adding additional orders (eg, laboratory tests, monitoring parameters) can redirect the order without having to cancel the ordering procedure.

The order entry system should be designed to bypass or transmit alert notification in electronic form without having to directly act on the alert at that moment. An ability to temporarily bypass a warning for a predetermined amount of time but still be able to present that same alert in the future is a desirable feature for a number of situations.[41] For example, it can be important for a consultant to send a message electronically to the primary care provider without having to alter care that is not desirable for the patient at that point in time.

EASE OF USE OF LINKS TO RESOURCES

Clinicians should have easy electronic access to supporting data for each order and alert. Hypertext links to authoritative online sources have been proposed as a method of supplementing information provided by commercial CDS software. Care must be taken to use reliable, stable, and trusted sources that meet standards set by the Health on the Net guidelines.[42]

The use of links to electronic resources available from the National Library of Medicine (NLM) is a source for authoritative information available provided at no cost to the consumer to assist with local hospital and health system CDS. Information from these types of sources is available from any computer connected to the Internet. NLM information is not included in commercial CDS programs, as they cannot be directly added for commercial use. However, links to these sources can be incorporated outside of commercial CDS systems into a local hospital and health system CDS.

National Library of Medicine Information

Information from the NLM includes DailyMed,[43] which is the official provider of FDA label information (package inserts). Information available includes the most current approved labeling for most prescription and many nonprescription drugs available. The Web page links at DailyMed are permanent, meaning that they will direct to the most current package insert material in use submitted to the FDA. DailyMed permanent links may include, for example, strengthened warnings undergoing FDA review or minor editorial changes. Although use of the official updated approved prescribing information from this site is invaluable, no decision support is provided by FDA labeling information. For example, if a drug pairing results in a potential interaction that should be avoided, the package insert will not recommend alternative drugs that might be more suitable. In addition, drug dosages and directions may not provide information on common use, as off-label (non-FDA–approved) use in specific populations, notably pediatric dosing, are omitted.

Patient Education

Additional information and handouts about medicine and disease states are available on NLM's site MedlinePlus Web.[44] This site also can be used as a portal for patient drug information handouts designed by The American Society of Health-System Pharmacists, Inc. These drug information sheets are available in a standard format, written at the eighth-grade reading level, and are also available in Spanish. The English sheet can be used to explain the Spanish sheet to a patient who is more comfortable with information in a native language.

Food and Drug Administration and Patient Safety

The FDA Web site includes a wide range of resources. The current and resolved drug shortage page[45] is valuable for maintaining order entry systems. Many order entry systems include links to allow barcoded medication administration (BCMA) using handheld devices, which can assist in accurately confirming that the right patient receives the right drug in the right dose by the right route at the right time. However products that are unavailable because of shortages may require local addition of alternative barcoded drugs to ensure proper scanning and documenting of drug items.[46] The FDA Web site can be used to verify the appropriate barcode values and formats to ensure proper scanning. Locally prepared items, such as intravenous admixtures specific to an institution, could be designed to be read by barcode readers during medication administration. Ensuring basic usability of BCMA items is critical to ensure timely drug administration and documentation, and to avoid potentially risky workarounds in medication administration.

Many FDA-approved drugs have significant risks that require education before and during use of selected high-risk drugs. The FDA Web site has updated, online links to Risk Evaluation and Mitigation Strategies (REMS), which may include Patient Medication Guides to inform and educate patients about the serious risk associated with selected drug treatments. These guidelines are available and can be searched at an online section of the FDA Web page.[47] Because information contained in individual REMS data sheets may change over time, and because patients should receive copies of REMS sheets with each drug with significant risks, a link to these sheets could be incorporated into the medication process and at the time of dispensing or discharge.

Clinical Trials

ClinicalTrials.gov[48] is a registry and results database of publicly and privately supported clinical studies of human participants conducted around the world. All interventional studies of drugs, biological products, or devices that are subject to FDA regulation have been required to list this information since 2007.[49] The Web site allows search by drug, condition, city, state, or country. Searching information that explains how to conduct both a basic and detailed search is available at that site to target studies of interest. Links to internal databases (intranet) for investigational study protocols can be added to allow practitioners access to data needed when deemed appropriate for patient use. Confidential information can be password protected.

Centers for Disease Control and Prevention

The Centers for Disease Control and Prevention (CDC) is the US health protection agency. The mission of the CDC is to protect America from health, safety, and security threats, both foreign and in the United States. The CDC Web site[50] provides current timely information on diseases and conditions, including advice on healthy living, traveler's heath, emergency preparedness recommendations, and vaccination information. Also available on the CDC site is a review of current and emerging disease states, in the Morbidity and Mortality Weekly Reports cases of notifiable reported diseases.[51]

National Guideline Clearinghouse

Although the use of private or individually maintained order sets was at one time promoted as a method of gaining clinician acceptance with electronic order entry development, they may not include accepted or cost-effective use of resources. To comply with meaningful use, treatments need to comply with accepted, published methods, including supporting references.[52] The National Guideline Clearinghouse[53] is a public resource for evidence-based clinical practice guidelines and recommendations from the Agency for Healthcare Research and Quality. Information from this site might be used to assist with development of local best practice guidelines and order sets designed to improve consistency and quality while reducing or maintaining cost.

ONCOLOGY-SPECIFIC ORDER SETS

Order sets are most useful where standard of care is well defined. Examples of settings in which order sets are may be useful include routine surgical procedures, oncology protocols, and investigational clinical trials. For surgical procedures, order sets can ensure that appropriate tests are ordered before surgery, that dietary restrictions before a scheduled procedure are timed, and that preoperative medications such as antibiotics or antiemetics can be scheduled with a few keystrokes. Oncology order protocols are highly standardized and may be dose based on laboratory values, height, weight, age, or calculations derived by any number of patient characteristics. In practice, oncology and investigational drug order sets may include orders for drugs that greatly exceed ranges set by commercial CDS systems. It is important that these orders are reviewed and approved in advance, and the CDS warnings are not displayed, which might lead to modification of established protocol dosing.

SUMMARY

As with all computer systems developed by groups that are not individual users, testing, managing, and maintaining of local CDS systems is a continuous requirement.[54] Feedback on nursing issues is most critical to ensure that unanswered needs are appropriately addressed. Nurses and advanced practice nurses should have an open line of communication with the information technology department in their facilities and continue with open dialogue to enhance and support computerized practitioner order entry and CDS system development and refinement, whether commercial or homegrown systems are used. The nurse is often the last safety defense for the patient in medication administration. Nurses must advocate for timely, manageable, safe, and accurate technology uses to facilitate their work with patients.

REFERENCES

1. HITECH Act Enforcement Interim Final Rule. U.S. Department of Health & Human Services. 2009. Available at: http://www.hhs.gov/ocr/privacy/hipaa/administrative/enforcementrule/hitechenforcementifr.html. Accessed January 25, 2015.
2. HealthIT.gov. Meaningful use definition and meaningful use objectives of EHRs. U.S. Department of Health and Human Services. 2014. Available at: www.healthit.gov/providers-professionals/meaningful-use-definition-objectives. Accessed January 26, 2015.
3. Centers for Medicare & Medicaid Services. Definition stage 1 of meaningful use. 2014. Available at: http://www.cms.gov/regulations-and-guidance/legislation/ehrincentiveprograms/meaningful_use.html. Accessed January 1, 2015.
4. Classen DC, Bates DW. Finding the meaning in meaningful use. N Engl J Med 2001;365:855–8. Available at: http://www.ncbi.nlm.nih.gov/pubmed/21879906. Accessed January 24, 2015.
5. Blumenthal D, Tavenner M. The 'meaningful use' regulation for electronic health records. N Engl J Med 2010;353:501–4. Available at: http://www.ncbi.nlm.nih.gov/pubmed/20647183. Accessed January 23, 2015.
6. Greenhalgh T, Potts HW, Wong G, et al. Tensions and paradoxes in electronic patient record research: a systematic literature review using the meta-narrative method. Millbank Q 2009;87(4):729–88. Available at: www.ncbi.nlm.nih.gov/pubmed/20021585. Accessed January 24, 2015.
7. Murphy J. The journey to meaningful use of electronic health records. Nurs Econ 2010;28(4):283–6. Available at: http://europepmc.org/abstract/med/21761616. Accessed January 21, 2015.
8. Sensmeier J. Alliance for Nursing Informatics statement to the Robert Wood Johnson Foundation Initiative on the Future of nursing: acute care, focusing on the area of technology, October 19, 2009. Comput Inform Nurs 2010;28(1):63–7. Available at: http://www.ncbi.nlm.nih.gov/pubmed/19940623. Accessed January 21, 2015.
9. Roshanov PS, Fernandes N, Wilczynski JM, et al. Features of effective computerised clinical decision support systems: meta-regression of 162 randomised trials. BMJ 2013;346:f657. Available at: http://www.ncbi.nlm.nih.gov/pubmed/23412440. Accessed January 21, 2015.
10. Kohn L, Corrigan J, Donaldson M. To err is human: building a safer health system. 2014. Available at: http://www.iom.edu/reports/1999/to-err-is-human-building-a-safer-health-system.aspx. Accessed January 26, 2015.
11. Barlas S. FDA weighs updating its bar-code mandate: hospital pharmacies worry about implementation. P T 2012;37(3):162–72. Available at: http://www.ncbi.nlm.nih.gov/pmc/articles/PMC3351875/. Accessed January 23, 2015.
12. Kuperman GJ, Reichley RM, Bailey TC. Using commercial knowledge bases for clinical decision support: opportunities, hurdles, and recommendations. J Am Med Inform Assoc 2006;13(4):369–71. Available at: http://www.ncbi.nlm.nih.gov/pmc/articles/PMC1513681/. Accessed January 25, 2015.
13. Hsieh TC, Kuperman GJ, Jaggi T, et al. Characteristics and consequences of drug allergy alert overrides in a computerized physician order entry system. J Am Med Inform Assoc 2004;11(6):482–91. Available at: http://www.ncbi.nlm.nih.gov/pubmed/15298998. Accessed January 23, 2015.
14. Parke C, Santiago E, Zussy B, et al. Reduction of clinical support warnings through recategorization of severity levels. Am J Health Syst Pharm 2015;72(2):144–8. Available at: http://www.ncbi.nlm.nih.gov/pubmed/25550138. Accessed January 24, 2015.

Clinical Decision Support **323**

15. Fox J, Thomson R. Clinical decision support systems: a discussion of quality, safety and legal liability issues. Proc AMIA Symp 2002;265–9. Available at: http://www.ncbi.nlm.nih.gov/pmc/articles/PMC2244432/. Accessed January 21, 2015.
16. Kesselheim AS, Cresswell K, Phansalkar S, et al. Clinical decision support systems could be modified to reduce 'alert fatigue' while still minimizing the risk of litigation. Health Aff (Millwood) 2011;30(12):2310–7. Available at: http://www.ncbi.nlm.nih.gov/pubmed/22147858. Accessed January 21, 2015.
17. Phansalkar S, Van der Sijs H, Tucker AD, et al. Drug-drug interactions that should be non-interruptive in order to reduce alert fatigue in electronic health records. J Am Med Inform Assoc 2013;20(3):489–93. Available at: http://www.ncbi.nlm.nih.gov/pmc/articles/PMC3628052/. Accessed January 21, 2015.
18. Phansalkar S, Desai AA, Bell D, et al. High-priority drug-drug interactions for use in electronic health records. J Am Med Inform Assoc 2012;19(5):735–43. Available at: http://www.ncbi.nlm.nih.gov/pmc/articles/PMC3422823/. Accessed January 22, 2015.
19. van der Weijden T, Boivin A, Burgers J, et al. Clinical practice guidelines and patient decision aids. An inevitable relationship. J Clin Epidemiol 2012;65(60): 584–9. Available at: http://www.ncbi.nlm.nih.gov/pubmed/22297117. Accessed January 23, 2015.
20. Ferranti JM, Horvath MM, Jansen J, et al. Using a computerized provider order entry system to meet the unique prescribing needs of children: description of an advanced dosing model. BMC Med Inform Decis Mak 2011;11:14. Available at: http://www.ncbi.nlm.nih.gov/pubmed/21338518. Accessed January 4, 2015.
21. Phansalkar S, Wright A, Kuperman GJ, et al. Towards meaningful medication-related clinical decision support: recommendations for an initial implementation. Appl Clin Inform 2011;2(1):50–62. Available at: http://www.ncbi.nlm.nih.gov/pubmed/23616860. Accessed January 22, 2015.
22. Russ AL, Zillich AJ, Mcmanus MS, et al. Prescribers' interactions with medication alerts at the point of prescribing: a multi-method, in situ investigation of the human-computer interaction. Int J Med Inform 2012;81(4):232–43. Available at: http://www.ncbi.nlm.nih.gov/pubmed/22296761. Accessed January 26, 2015.
23. Phansalkar S, Zachariah M, Seidling HM, et al. Evaluation of medication alerts in electronic health records for compliance with human factors principles. J Am Med Inform Assoc 2014;21(e2):e332–40. Available at: http://www.ncbi.nlm.nih.gov/pubmed/24780721. Accessed January 25, 2015.
24. Jarzyna D, Jungquist CR, Pasero C, et al. American Society for Pain Management nursing guidelines on monitoring for opioid-induced sedation and respiratory depression. Pain Manag Nurs 2011;12(3):118–45.e10. Available at: http://www.ncbi.nlm.nih.gov/pubmed/21893302. Accessed January 23, 2015.
25. Fields L. DNR does not mean no care. J Neurosci Nurs 2007;39(5):294–6. Available at: http://www.ncbi.nlm.nih.gov/pubmed/17966296. Accessed January 25, 2015.
26. Blanco-reina E, Ariza-zafra G, Ocaña-riola R, et al. 2012 American Geriatrics Society Beers criteria: enhanced applicability for detecting potentially inappropriate medications in European older adults? A comparison with the Screening Tool of Older Person's Potentially Inappropriate Prescriptions. J Am Geriatr Soc 2014; 62(7):1217–23. Available at: http://www.ncbi.nlm.nih.gov/pubmed/24917083. Accessed January 19, 2015.
27. Brouwer RM, Follath F, Bühler FR. Review of the cardiovascular adversity of the calcium antagonist beta-blocker combination: implications for antihypertensive

therapy. J Cardiovasc Pharmacol 1985;7(Suppl 4):S38–44. Available at: http://www.ncbi.nlm.nih.gov/pubmed/2412010. Accessed January 23, 2015.

28. Allen R, O'Brien BM. Uses of misoprostol in obstetrics and gynecology. Rev Obstet Gynecol 2009;2(3):159–68. Available at: http://www.ncbi.nlm.nih.gov/pmc/articles/PMC2760893/. Accessed January 25, 2015.

29. Vaccine information for adults. Centers for Disease Control and Prevention. 2014. Available at: http://www.cdc.gov/vaccines/adults/rec-vac/pregnant.html. Accessed January 27, 2015.

30. Fayssoil A, Issi J, Guerbaa M, et al. Torsade de pointes induced by citalopram and amiodarone. Ann Cardiol Angeiol (Paris) 2011;60(3):165–8. Available at: http://www.ncbi.nlm.nih.gov/pubmed/21295285. Accessed January 23, 2015.

31. Kannankeril PJ, Roden DM. Drug-induced long QT and torsade de pointes: recent advances. Curr Opin Cardiol 2007;22(1):39–43. Available at: http://www.ncbi.nlm.nih.gov/pubmed/17143043. Accessed January 13, 2015.

32. Drew BJ, Ackerman MJ, Funk M, et al. Prevention of torsade de pointes in hospital settings: a scientific statement from the American Heart Association and the American College of Cardiology Foundation. J Am Coll Cardiol 2010;55(9): 934–47. Available at: http://www.ncbi.nlm.nih.gov/pmc/articles/PMC3057430/. Accessed January 20, 2015.

33. Husch M, Sullivan C, Rooney D, et al. Insights from the sharp end of intravenous medication errors: implications for infusion pump technology. Qual Saf Health Care 2005;14(2):80–6. Available at: http://www.ncbi.nlm.nih.gov/pmc/articles/PMC1743987/. Accessed February 3, 2015.

34. Kuperman GJ, Bobb A, Payne TH, et al. Medication-related clinical decision support in computerized provider order entry systems: a review. J Am Med Inform Assoc 2007;14(1):29–40. Available at: http://www.ncbi.nlm.nih.gov/pmc/articles/PMC2215064/.

35. Poissant L, Pereira J, Tamblyn R, et al. The impact of electronic health records on time efficiency of physicians and nurses: a systematic review. J Am Med Inform Assoc 2005;12(5):505–16. Available at: http://www.ncbi.nlm.nih.gov/pmc/articles/PMC1205599/. Accessed January 23, 2015.

36. Yeung MS, Lapinsky SE, Granton JT, et al. Examining nursing vital signs documentation workflow: barriers and opportunities in general internal medicine units. J Clin Nurs 2012;21(7–8):975–82. Available at: http://www.ncbi.nlm.nih.gov/pubmed/22243491. Accessed January 23, 2015.

37. UMLS - LOINC. US National Library of Medicine. 2010. Available at: http://www.nlm.nih.gov/research/umls/loinc_main.html. Accessed January 26, 2015.

38. SNOMED Clinical Terms® (SNOMED CT®). US National Library of Medicine. 2009. Available at: http://www.nlm.nih.gov/research/umls/Snomed/snomed_main.html. Accessed January 26, 2015.

39. ICD-9-CM and ICD-10. Centers for Medicare & Medicaid Services. 2014. Available at: http://www.cms.gov/Medicare/Coding/ICD9ProviderDiagnosticCodes/index.html. Accessed January 21, 2015.

40. Karnes JH, Van driest S, Bowton EA, et al. Using systems approaches to address challenges for clinical implementation of pharmacogenomics. Wiley Interdiscip Rev Syst Biol Med 2014;6(2):125–35. Available at: http://www.ncbi.nlm.nih.gov/pubmed/24319008. Accessed January 23, 2015.

41. Wright A, Phansalkar S, Bloomrosen M, et al. Best practices in clinical decision support: the case of preventive care reminders. Appl Clin Inform 2010;1:331–45. Available at: http://www.ncbi.nlm.nih.gov/pmc/articles/mid/NIHMS318270/. Accessed February 3, 2015.

42. About Health On the Net (HON): background. About Health On the Net (HON): background. 1997. Available at: http://www.hon.ch/global/index.html; http://www.hon.ch/HONcode/Conduct.html. Accessed January 27, 2015.
43. About DailyMed. DailyMed. National Library of Medicine. Available at: http://dailymed.nlm.nih.gov/dailymed/about-dailymed.cfm. Accessed January 26, 2015.
44. Medicines: MedlinePlus. US National Library of Medicine. 2015. Available at: http://www.nlm.nih.gov/medlineplus/medicines.html. Accessed January 27, 2015.
45. FDA. FDA drug shortages. U.S. Department of Health and Human Services. Available at: http://www.accessdata.fda.gov/scripts/drugshortages/default.cfm. Accessed January 27, 2015.
46. Koppel R, Wetterneck T, Telles JL, et al. Workarounds to barcode medication administration systems: their occurrences, causes, and threats to patient safety. J Am Med Inform Assoc 2008;15(4):408–23. Available at: http://www.ncbi.nlm.nih.gov/pmc/articles/PMC2442264/. Accessed January 27, 2015.
47. Approved Risk Evaluation and Mitigation Strategies (REMS). Available at: http://www.fda.gov/Drugs/DrugSafety/PostmarketDrugSafetyInformationforPatientsand Providers/ucm111350.htm or http://www.fda.gov/Drugs/DrugSafety/Postmarket DrugSafetyInformationforPatientsandProviders/ucm111350.htm#Current. Accessed January 28, 2015.
48. Clinical Trials. U.S. National Institutes of Health. Available at: www.clinicaltrials.gov. Accessed January 24, 2015.
49. ClinicalTrials.gov and FDAAA - Frequently Asked Questions. National Institutes of Health. 2011. Available at: http://grants.nih.gov/clinicaltrials_fdaaa/faq.htm. Accessed January 27, 2015.
50. Centers for Disease Control and Prevention. Available at: http://www.cdc.gov/. Accessed January 23, 2015.
51. Morbidity and Mortality Weekly Report (MMWR) Centers for Disease Control and Prevention. 2015. Available at: http://www.cdc.gov/mmwr/. Accessed January 13, 2015.
52. ISMP's Guidelines for Standard Order Sets. Institute for Safe Medication Practices. 2010. Available at: http://www.ismp.org/tools/guidelines/standardordersets.pdf. Accessed January 24, 2015.
53. National Guideline Clearinghouse. Agency for Healthcare Research and Quality. 2014. Available at: http://www.guideline.gov/index.aspx. Accessed January 23, 2015.
54. Bates DW, Kuperman GJ, Wang S, et al. Ten commandments for effective clinical decision support: making the practice of evidence-based medicine a reality. J Am Med Inform Assoc 2003;10(6):523–30. Available at: http://www.ncbi.nlm.nih.gov/pmc/articles/PMC264429/. Accessed January 21, 2015.

Utilization of Clinical Practice Guidelines

Barriers and Facilitators

Melanie R. Keiffer, DNP, ANP-BC, CCRN[a,b,*]

KEYWORDS

- Clinical practice guidelines • Nurse practitioners • Electronic health record
- Clinical decision support tool • Patient safety

KEY POINTS

- Clinical practice guidelines are tools used to assist health care professionals in clinical decision making with the ultimate goal of improving patient care.
- Promoting the implementation of clinical practice guidelines at the point of care delivery is a hurdle to translating scientific findings into practice.
- As access to electronic evidence sources increase, the amount of evidence available to clinicians for clinical decision support is overwhelming.
- Increased adoption of electronic health records and clinical decision support tools will move clinical practice guidelines more rapidly to the patient encounter.

UTILIZATION OF CLINICAL PRACTICE GUIDELINES: BARRIERS AND FACILITATORS

Clinical practice guidelines are designed to improve quality of care, reduce variation in practice and ensure evidence-based care is delivered when appropriate. Despite the creation of guidelines at national and international levels, guidelines are underutilized by clinicians at the bedside to improve patient care. Clinical practice guidelines are "systematically developed statements to assist practitioners and patients to make decisions about appropriate health care for specific circumstances."[1(p13)] In the United States, the National Guideline Clearinghouse, a public database of evidence-based clinical practice guidelines, provides clinicians with a method to advance excellence in care by decreasing the gap between evidence and practice. Although high-quality, well-developed, clinical practice guidelines are available, these tools are only useful if implemented locally to improve patient care.

Disclosure: None.

[a] College of Nursing and Health, Madonna University, 36600 Schoolcraft Road, Livonia, MI 48150, USA; [b] Advanced Practice Provider Services, Henry Ford West Bloomfield Hospital, 6777 West Maple Road, West Bloomfield Township, MI 48322, USA

* College of Nursing and Health, Madonna University, 36600 Schoolcraft Road, Livonia, MI 48150.

E-mail address: keiffermelanie@gmail.com

Nurs Clin N Am 50 (2015) 327–345
http://dx.doi.org/10.1016/j.cnur.2015.03.007
0029-6465/15/$ – see front matter © 2015 Elsevier Inc. All rights reserved.

nursing.theclinics.com

Translating evidence into practice while implementing, planning, and caring for patients is a core competency of nurse practitioners and physician assistants in acute care settings. The term "advanced practice provider" has been used to describe nurse practitioners and physician assistants who provide care to acute and critically ill patients. These advanced practice providers have the expertise to guide the process change necessary to bring clinical practice guidelines to the bedside to improve health and safety for patients, as well as the quality of care. The perception and use of clinical practice guidelines with this health care provider population is poorly understood. The majority of research on the development, implementation, and use of clinical practice guidelines is focused on physician behavior.[2] Further research exploring the attitudes, knowledge, and behaviors of nurse practitioners and physician assistants toward the use of clinical guidelines is needed to identify what facilitators and barriers exist. Understanding these perceptions is a key to engaging advanced practice providers in the creation, implementation, and ongoing surveillance of clinical practice guidelines pertinent to their patient population.

STATEMENT OF THE PROBLEM

Decisions about when, why, and how to pursue certain diagnoses and treatments are complicated. Patient care interventions are based on scientific principles, theoretical knowledge, and a clinician's expertise. Clinical practice guidelines exist as tools to augment clinician decision making, yet several barriers to implementation have been identified in the literature. Researchers cite a lack of knowledge of guideline existence, complexity of guidelines, staff attitude, lack of training, time, and resource constraints as reasons for nonadherence to clinical practice guidelines.[3-5] Clinicians are encouraged to use evidence-based clinical practice guidelines in light of available resources and circumstances presented by individual patients to provide the current standard of care. Traditionally, "standard of care" has been defined as "the level at which the average, prudent provider in a given community would practice."[6] Specialty societies, health plans, accrediting organizations, private organizations, and federal agencies such as the Agency for Healthcare Research and Quality are now setting, modifying, monitoring, and publicizing standards of care for patients. Potential liability exists for the clinician who does not follow the minimal acceptable level of care determined by consensus of providers, consumers, or these outside agencies. Buppert[7] suggests the standard of care address the following questions:

- Did the clinician do the right thing at the right time?
- Was effective care provided to the patient?
- Was care provided safely and in an appropriate time frame?
- Was the outcome as good as expected, given the patient's condition, personal characteristics, and the current state of medical science?

Clinicians may be more likely to adopt clinical practice guidelines if they believe guidelines offer malpractice litigation protection and support a standard of care. Utilization of clinical practice guidelines is one method to facilitate clinical decision making in providing safer, quality care to patients. Yet, some clinicians believe guidelines characterize a rigid or oversimplified practice of medicine and refer to guidelines as "cookbook medicine." At the community hospital setting for this project, clinician utilization of clinical practice guidelines to guide complex clinical decision making was unknown.

PURPOSE

The purpose of this project was to seek an understanding of what factors promote or prevent the implementation of evidence-based clinical practice guidelines at the point of care delivery using a population of neuroscience advanced practice providers.

BACKGROUND

Even with the exponential growth of publicly available clinical practice guidelines, ease of access to high-quality evidence is out of reach for many clinicians. As access to electronic evidence sources increases, the amount of evidence available to clinicians for clinical decision support is overwhelming. It is often difficult for providers to stay current with the evidence necessary to provide the standard of care. In practice, clinicians use experience, education, literature, a patient's preference, and clinical data to make clinical decisions. Patient interventions may be adopted widely but not necessarily based on evidence. Clinical practice guidelines are useful mechanisms to break down complex datasets into more manageable pieces, promoting the effective use of evidence for busy clinicians to individualize patient care.

Despite immediate clinical practice guideline availability in this technological era, use of practice guidelines varies widely. Dissemination of new information is haphazard and inconsistent, and the impact on treatment decisions for care is unknown. Previously, a 17-year time-frame was estimated to incorporate evidence into clinical practice.[8] Despite the availability of evidence at the point of care and clinical practice guidelines embedded in the electronic health record, the dynamic workflow of a clinician's use of guidelines in practice is poorly understood.[9] At the clinical site, one process amenable to the use of guidelines was analyzed in an attempt to understand the impact of clinical practice guidelines in clinician decision making (**Fig. 1**).

In the community hospital where this project was undertaken, the patient with intracranial hemorrhage owing to anticoagulation is among the highest acuity patients on the neuroscience service. As clinicians caring for patients with this devastating complication, use of evidence-based treatment recommendations to guide treatment is crucial to patient safety. The decision to reverse anticoagulants is made by the clinician after consideration of intended benefit and potential risks to the patient. This diagnosis was selected purposefully for evaluation at the clinical site because anticoagulated patients have a greater risk of hematoma expansion, and subsequent clinical deterioration and death, necessitating vigorous reversal of coagulopathy.[10] Because management of anticoagulation-associated intracranial hemorrhage prompts urgent reversal of anticoagulants with variable treatment options, an evidence-based anticoagulation reversal guideline is available at the clinical site. The locally developed guidelines serve as a guide to select initial doses and agents once appropriate patients are selected. As one of the most difficult patients for the clinician to treat, understanding of barrier and facilitators to use of the guideline is helpful.

The advanced practice provider is among the first caregivers to arrive at the bedside of the intracranial hemorrhage patient; the neurosurgeon or neurointensivist may not be available immediately. The advanced practice provider initiates the care management of this patient by assessing, diagnosing, and writing anticoagulation reversal orders. Although intracerebral hemorrhage represents only 10% to 15% of all cerebrovascular events, it is associated with substantial morbidity and mortality for patients.[11] The incidence of oral anticoagulation-associated intracerebral hemorrhage is growing owing to the increasing use of warfarin, the emergence of multiple new blood thinners, and the older age of treated patients.[12] Optimal treatment is yet to be defined, making this a complex patient to manage. In the absence of well-designed, randomized, controlled trials, treatment of this patient varies widely.[10,11] Experts agree reversal

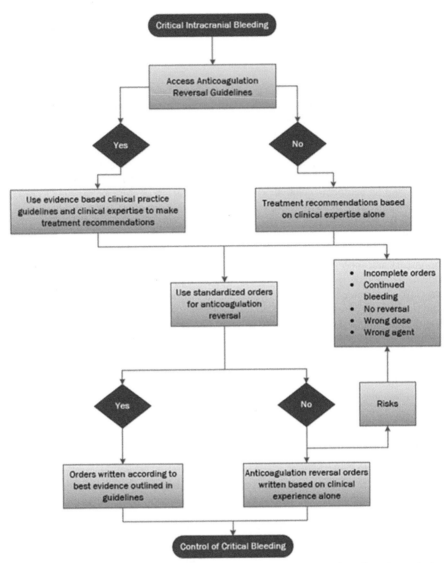

Fig. 1. Failure mode effects analysis (FMEA) of use of locally developed anticoagulation reversal guidelines for patients with anticoagulation related intracranial hemorrhage.

of anticoagulation without delay is necessary to prevent hematoma expansion during the initial 24 to 48 hours.[13]

An evaluation tool recommended to identify and prevent process problems is failure mode and effects analysis. This prospective risk assessment process is designed to identify and prevent process problems before they occur.[14] To assess risk in relation to adherence to the anticoagulation guideline, the American Hospital Association and Institute for Safe Medication Practices recommend analysis of the prescribing phase, order processing phase and medication dispensing phase.[15] Because nonadherence to practice guidelines may jeopardize patient safety or result in medication errors, risk assessment is 1 method used to evaluate error-prone processes. Failure mode and effects analysis reveals multiple potential failure modes owing to a lack of advanced practice provider utilization of the anticoagulation reversal guidelines (**Table 1**).

SIGNIFICANCE OF THE PROBLEM
Health care

The Institute of Medicine's *Promoting Adoption of Clinical Practice Guidelines* report challenges the health care community to create systems from within that promote

Table 1		
Failure mode and effects analysis implementation of anticoagulation reversal guidelines		
Process and Sub-processes	**Potential Failure Modes**	**Effects**
Prescribing		
Assess patient	PMH not readily available	Clinical situation not considered (renal, liver function, allergies, concomitant use of other drugs)
	Medication reconciliation incomplete	Risk for choice of wrong reversal agent
	Allergies not documented clearly or accurately	Allergic response
Monitoring effects of medication	Laboratory data results insufficient, insufficient monitoring, wrong tests ordered	Delay in treatment, wrong treatment, failure to recognize consequences before harm occur, no achievement of pharmacologic reversal
Choice of correct agent	Wrong agent selected Provider unaware of availability of treatment guidelines for anticoagulation reversal	No reversal, continuation of major bleeding
Order processing		
Standard order sets	Providers unaware of standard order sets	Incomplete orders Delay in treatment Wrong treatment
Timely delivery and administration	Not ordering stat Inaccurate order entry	Delay in distribution of medication
Use of anticoagulation guidelines	Lack of advanced practice provider competency and education on anticoagulation guidelines, lack of familiarity with content, complexity in guidelines	Overdose, underdose, failure to recognize adverse effects
Medication dispensing		
Use of guidelines by interdisciplinary team	Failure to communicate with interdisciplinary team, attending staff physicians, consultants, pharmacy, nursing Staff attitudes and belief in validity of guidelines	Delay in treatment, wrong treatment, failure to recognize consequences before harm occur, no achievement of pharmacologic reversal

the uptake and use of clinical practice guidelines at the point of care.[16] The Institute of Medicine recognizes this as one of the main steps in translating research findings into the mainstream of practice. A growing body of evidence shows that the rate of clinical practice guideline adoption is affected by the interaction of the guideline users (physicians, nurses, pharmacists), the characteristics of the guideline (eg, ease of use, strength of the evidence) and the context of practice (eg, inpatient, ambulatory).[17] Efficient and effective guidelines impact patient safety and quality by increasing the consistency of behavior and replacing idiosyncratic behaviors with best practices. Increased adoption of electronic health records and clinical decision support tools will move clinical practice guidelines more rapidly to the patient encounter. These practices standardize and improve the quality of care by reducing errors.[18] Use of electronic health record clinical decision support tools is shown to improve patient safety.[19]

Advanced Practice Nursing

Translating evidence into practice while implementing, planning, and caring for patients is one of the core competencies of nurse practitioners and physician assistants.[20,21] The role of the nurse practitioner is to generate knowledge from clinical practice to improve practice and patient outcomes by analyzing clinical guidelines for individualized application into practice.[21] Advanced practice nurses have the ability to translate scientific knowledge quickly and effectively to benefit patients in the daily demands of practice environments. Practice guidelines enhance clinician decision making by clearly describing and appraising the scientific evidence and reasoning behind clinical recommendations. Critically appraised and synthesized evidence is fundamental to quality practice. Understanding the barriers and facilitators to use of clinical practice guidelines by this population is a precursor to understanding use of clinical practice guidelines and ultimately improving patient care.

IMPACT OF PROJECT ON POPULATION

Adherence to well-designed clinical practice guidelines is recognized as a strategy to reduce error and improve outcomes for neuroscience patients. Neurosurgical and cerebrovascular adverse events such as thromboembolic events, infection, wrong level surgery, management of vasospasm, and salt wasting syndromes are complications likely be reduced by use of evidence-based guidelines and protocols.[22] In recent years, professional medical and nursing organizations attempted to monitor effects on practice by endorsing clinical practice guidelines on association websites. Successful efforts to evaluate clinical practice guidelines by the American Association of Neurologic Surgeons and the Congress of Neurologic Surgeons resulted in systematic approaches to cervical spine injury, concussion, and severe traumatic brain injury.[23] The American Association of Neuroscience Nurses grants free access to electronic clinical practice guidelines to assist nurses in delivering optimum quality-focused patient care to specific neuroscience patient populations.[24] Using expert consensus guidelines to develop protocols, order sets, clinical algorithms, and clinical decision support tools is recommended to shorten the time frame to translate evidence into practice.[25]

Despite the availability of electronic access to evidence based resources at the clinical site, it was unknown to what extent clinicians in this project setting use them to deliver care. The clinical site for this scholarly project was a 200-bed community hospital in an academic health system with electronic access to clinical practice guidelines to enhance clinician decision making. Data were gathered on the use of clinical practice guidelines to support the anecdotal notion that the neuroscience advanced practice providers were unfamiliar with guidelines specific to the patient population. The survey assessed the extent to which clinicians agree with and trust clinical practice guidelines, the clarity and ease of use, and the extent of use with a specific patient population. Results from the survey provided valuable insight to develop education and process improvement and to expand access and use of evidence based guidelines at the clinical site.

APPLICATION OF THEORETIC FRAMEWORK

Although clinical practice guidelines encourage the consistent, efficient application of evidence when used by clinicians at the bedside, a knowledge translation gap exists.[25] Social, cognitive, and motivational factors enable efficient knowledge translation in an organization.[25] The interrelationship between several concepts impacts the utilization of clinical practice guidelines in clinical practice (**Fig. 2**).

The literature reveals many barriers and facilitators that impede the successful implementation of clinical practice guidelines. Understanding of individual predisposition to change and the optimal approaches to change clinician's behavior is incomplete. More theory-based study is needed to better inform the design of interventions to implement successfully evidenced-based findings in complex organizations. Individual professional decisions are central to the execution of clinical practice guidelines. It is useful to observe stimuli and responses in real-world situations to understand the human mechanisms necessary to improve behavior change strategies.[26] In social cognitive theory, Bandura[27] proposes that people regulate their own motivation within a network of interacting influences. Social cognitive theory describes a dynamic, ongoing process in which personal, environmental, and human behavior factors exert influence upon each other (**Fig. 3**). The survey assesses the impact of the hospital environment, peers, and self-motivation in the use of clinical practice guidelines in the population of neuroscience advanced practice providers.

Nevid[28] explains that social cognitive theory illustrates that individuals do not simply respond to environmental influences, but actively seek and interpret information. Because people, and not guidelines, are the agents of change, social cognitive theory provides understanding to the motivation of advanced practice providers in using clinical practice guidelines (**Fig. 4**). Social cognitive theory provides the feedback necessary for the implementation of best practice change process to occur. This theory was central to understanding and predicting clinicians' intentions and behaviors in the use to clinical practice guidelines. Assessing the core elements of the theory, implications for advanced practice that encourage rapid translation of evidence into practice are developed.

METHODOLOGY
Project Design

The purpose of this project was to assess factors that negatively or positively influenced advanced practice provider utilization of clinical practice guidelines in a community hospital. The method in this project was described in both a broad and narrow context relevant to neuroscience advanced practice provider clinical practice. A nonexperimental, cross-sectional, descriptive design was used to gather qualitative and quantitative data via survey. The project was approved by the institutional review boards at the project setting and the home university before survey distribution.

The survey was distributed to a convenience sample of all nurse practitioners and physician assistants working on a neuroscience specialty service at a community hospital. As clinicians responsible for health care delivery at the bedside, these advanced practice providers were chosen because they have the potential to narrow the gap that exists between standard of care and that which is actually delivered to patients

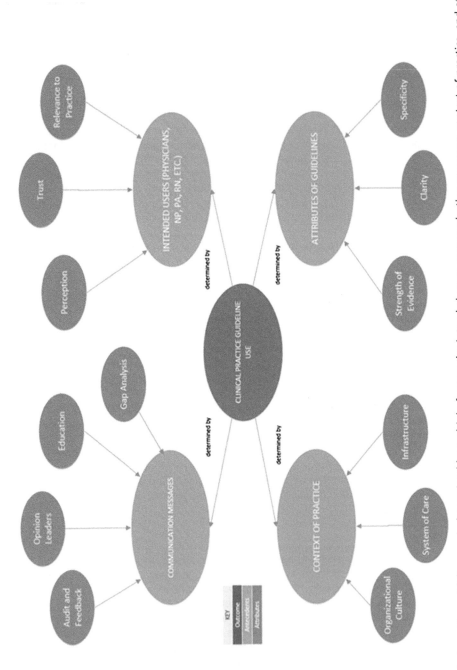

Fig. 2. Clinical practice guideline use is determined by multiple factors: the intended users, communication messages, context of practice, and attributes of the guidelines themselves.

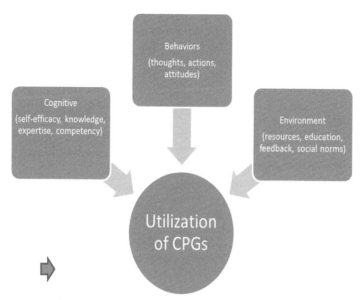

Fig. 3. Social cognitive theory explains the interaction between cognitive factors, environmental factors and behaviors in relation to use of clinical practice guidelines. (*Data from* Bandura A. A social cognitive theory of personality. In: Pervin L, John O, editors. Handbook of personality. 2nd edition. New York: Guilford Publications; 1999. p. 154–96.)

at this community hospital. Twenty-three credentialed nurse practitioner and physician assistant staff working full time, part time, or contingent on the neuroscience service were included in the survey population. Advanced practice providers currently in orientation, as well as advanced practice provider students and contingent employees who work less than 36 hours per month on the service were excluded. Recruitment of potential subjects was aided by the Neuroscience advanced practice provider team leader and the health system clinical coordinator.

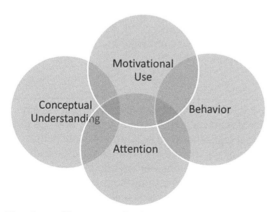

Fig. 4. Social cognitive theory illustrates individuals do not simply respond to environmental influences but actively seek and interpret information. People, not guidelines, are the agents of change. (*Data from* Bandura A. A social cognitive theory of personality. In: Pervin L, John O, editors. Handbook of personality. 2nd edition. New York: Guilford Publications; 1999. p. 154–96.)

The setting for the scholarly project was the neuroscience service of a 200-bed suburban community hospital, which is part of a 7-hospital urban health system. The primary condition reviewed was the acute management of patients with anticoagulation-related intracranial hemorrhage in a community hospital. Understanding internal and external factors that impact the use of evidence-based recommendations by advance practice providers for this high-acuity population was unknown. The rationale for surveying this group of advanced practice providers was to better understand what education and strategies might be used to facilitate use of clinical practice guidelines in the practice environment.

Data Collection Tool: Technology

The survey tool was designed with statements and open-ended questions to assess mechanisms that influence utilization of clinical practice guidelines. The tool was developed using a framework originally designed to assess a variety of barriers related to knowledge, attitudes and behaviors of practitioners toward clinical practice guidelines.[29] A second instrument describing attitudinal statements about a Centers for Disease Control and Prevention hand hygiene guideline was modified to fit the scholarly project setting.[30] A 4-point Likert-type scale ranging from strongly agree to strongly disagree was used to extract a positive or negative response. Eliminating the neutral response elicited a more discriminating and thoughtful response. The scale was 1 (strongly disagree), 2 (disagree), 3 (agree), and 4 (strongly agree). The survey was purposefully designed with both positive and negative wording to encourage respondents to read questions carefully. Part 1 was developed with 17 statements used as a general tool to assess attitudes toward any clinical practice guideline. Part 2 used 13 statements to assess heath system specific anticoagulation reversal guidelines. In addition, the tool asked 6 open-ended questions to obtain qualitative data about guideline knowledge and barriers and facilitators to using the specific guideline. Face validity was sought through doctorally prepared faculty evaluation and pilot survey. A pilot survey was completed by 2 acute care nurse practitioners who addressed ease of use, clarity, and the amount of time needed for completion.

The technology used in this project included an online survey system and the hospital email system. The survey was created using Qualtrics survey system and distributed via the project site employee e-mail system. Qualtrics, a secure, web-based software tool provided online reporting and data manipulation, functionality, and data export to Excel. Anonymity was ensured through the Qualtrics secure database by deidentification of respondents.

Data Analysis

Data gathered included demographic data of survey participants (**Table 2**). Demographics, use of clinical practice guidelines in general, and use of a hospital-specific anticoagulation reversal guideline. Of the 23 potential subjects, 17 (74%) completed the survey. The survey assessed the core concepts of knowledge, behaviors, and environmental factors impacting whether or not clinical practice guidelines were used. Attributes of the guidelines and knowledge of evidence based recommendations for acute management of patients with anticoagulation-related intracranial hemorrhage were assessed. Data were analyzed using the descriptive statistics procedure in Excel to determine and measure frequencies and central tendencies.

Qualitative data analysis was performed on open-ended questions by review of written narrative to identify themes and patterns in the data. The data were interpreted and applied in the context of the clinical question and concepts as outcomes. The meaning

Table 2
Demographics

	Frequency	Percent
Provider role		
Nurse practitioner	11	65
Physician assistant	6	35
Experience in neuroscience field (y)		
<5	8	47
6–10	5	29
11–20	4	24
Level of education		
Master of science	7	41
Master of science-nursing	9	53
Doctor of nursing practice	1	6
Current employment status		
Full time	14	82
Contingent	3	18

in the data was interpreted to ascertain what changes are necessary to improve practice (**Table 3**).

RESULTS

In assessing advanced practice provider use of clinical practice guidelines, statements and open-ended questions related to knowledge, attitude, and behaviors were evaluated via survey. Frequency distribution tables of results were constructed for both clinical practice guidelines in general and the hospital specific anticoagulation reversal guidelines (**Tables 2** and **4**). An overall response rate to determine the score and mean related to all the statements was calculated. Before computing the mean of the series of questions, negatively worded questions were assigned an opposite number of points than the positively worded questions. A higher score indicated fewer perceived barriers. A subscale mean response was calculated for statements relating to general clinical practice guideline adherence versus hospital-specific guideline adherence. Overall, 81% of the advanced practice providers surveyed perceived facilitators of clinical practice guidelines in general (**Fig. 5**) and 89% of advanced practice providers perceived facilitators of hospital specific anticoagulation reversal guidelines (**Fig. 6**).

The primary facilitators influencing the respondents to use clinical practice guidelines included:

- Patient care is standardized
- Patient outcomes are optimized
- Guidelines are practical to use
- Clinicians are familiar with guidelines in the neuroscience field
- Guidelines are readily accessible.

Five primary facilitators for using the hospital specific anticoagulation guidelines were similar:

- Patient care is standardized
- Patient outcomes are improved

Table 3
Survey responses to clinical practice guidelines in general (n = 17)

Facilitators (Descending Score)	SA (4), %	A (3), %	D (2), %	SD (1), %
Familiar with guidelines	18	70	12	0
Readily accessible	6	65	29	0
Practical to use	6	82	12	0
Facility places importance	12	47	35	6
Optimizes patient outcomes	12	82	12	0
Standardizes care	12	88	0	0
Sufficient administrative support/resources	0	59	35	6
Patient awareness	0	6	76	18
Protection from malpractice	0	65	35	0

Barriers (Ascending Score)	SA (1), %	SD (2), %	D (3), %	SD (4), %
Impossible to keep up guidelines	12	41	41	6
Too prescriptive	0	29	65	6
Cumbersome and inconvenient	0	12	82	6
Difficult to apply/adapt to practice	0	12	82	6
Cost outweighs benefit	0	24	76	0
Interfere with professional autonomy	0	18	76	6
Knowledge and creativity result in better patient outcomes	0	18	70	12
Use of guidelines optional in current employment	0	24	65	12

Negatively worded questions assigned the opposite number of points than positively worded questions. Barriers scoring scale: strongly agree = 1, agree = 2, disagree = 3, strongly disagree = 4. Facilitators scoring scale: strongly agree = 4, agree = 3, disagree = 2, strongly disagree=1. A higher score is associated with fewer perceived barriers in the use of clinical practice guidelines.
Abbreviations: A, agree; D, disagree; SA, strongly agree; SD, strongly disagree.

- Guidelines are practical to use
- Relevant to the neuroscience patient population
- Management expectation the use of guidelines

The only barrier that elicited a strong response (>50% agree/strongly agree) was the statement, "It is impossible to keep up with clinical practice guidelines in my field."

DISCUSSION
Relationship of Results to Framework

Individual professional decisions were central to the execution of clinical practice guidelines, understanding perceptions to similar clinical scenarios of patients encountered on a daily basis were integral to recommending approaches to improve adherence. Responses to open-ended questions regarding these high-acuity scenarios were evaluated to attain insight into factors that promote or prevent adherence to the use of clinical practice guidelines. Striking similarities in correct responses of complex treatment plans were noted in all 3 scenarios, demonstrating widespread use of the hospital-specific anticoagulation reversal protocol.

From the respondents' perspective, standardizing patient care and improving patient outcomes were the leading reasons to use clinical practice guidelines. Results

Table 4
Survey responses to health system specific AC reversal clinical practice guidelines ($n = 17$)

Facilitators (Descending Score)	SA (4), %	A (3), %	D (2), %	SD (1), %
Familiar with AC reversal guidelines	18	53	29	0
Knows how to access AC guidelines	18	53	29	0
Familiar with standard electronic order sets	12	65	23	0
Agree with guideline content	23	65	12	0
AC guidelines improve patient outcomes	29	65	6	0
AC guideline standardize patient care	23	76	0	0
Practical to use	23	71	6	0
Neurosurgeon/intensivist expectation	35	53	12	0
Manager expectation	29	65	6	0
Guideline relevant to patient population	41	53	6	0
Confidence in guideline developers	35	53	6	6
Responsibility of nurse practitioner/ physician assistant to order AC reversal and monitor	18	82	0	0
Barriers (Ascending Score)	**SA (1), %**	**A (2), %**	**D (3), %**	**SD (4), %**
Reversal guideline is difficult to apply	0	18	59	23

Negatively worded questions are assigned the opposite number of points than positively worded questions. Barriers scoring scale: strongly agree = 1, agree = 2, disagree = 3, strongly disagree = 4. Facilitators scoring scale: strongly agree = 4, agree = 3, disagree = 2, strongly disagree = 1. A higher score is associated with fewer perceived barriers in the use of clinical practice guidelines.

Abbreviations: A, agree; AC, anticoagulation; D, disagree; SA, strongly agree; SD, strongly disagree.

revealed numerous facilitators promoting successful implementation of clinical practice guidelines and few barriers. Using direct quotes, the core elements of the social cognitive theory were examined to develop implications for advanced practice that encourage rapid translation of evidence into practice.

Utilization of Clinical Practice Guidelines

■ Perceive Facilitators to Use ■ Perceive Barriers to Use

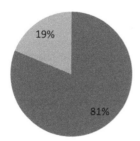

Fig. 5. Calculated overall response rate to survey part 1 (clinical practice guidelines in general) based on scores and means related to all statements. Negatively worded questions were assigned opposite number of points than the positively worded questions. Higher scores indicated fewer perceived barriers.

Utilization of Health System Anticoagulation Reversal Guidelines

■ Perceive Facilitators to Use   ■ Perceive Barriers to Use

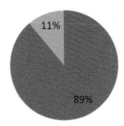

Fig. 6. Calculated overall response rate to survey part 2 (health system anticoagulation reversal guidelines) based on scores and means related to all statements. Negatively worded questions were assigned opposite number of points than the positively worded questions. Higher scores indicated fewer perceived barriers.

Behavioral Factors

Self-reported behavioral factors, such as thoughts, actions, and attitudes, were examined for perceptions that influence participants use of guidelines. Respondents cited the need for patient safety and acuity as factors that influenced the use of the guideline, "patient safety, I want to double check that I am doing the reversal correctly as we do not use these medications on a frequent basis, it is a safe way to provide care and maintain standards." Attributes of the guidelines also influenced use—"ease of use, consistency" and "I know the guideline is evidence based." Patient acuity status was addressed with "the seriousness of the diagnosis impacts my use" and "I want to be able to assess risk versus benefit of my plan." A strong sense of self-efficacy was present; some clinicians initiated behaviors necessary to attain the competency required to manage prospective situations, "I use the guideline all the time" and "I pull up the guidelines, print, read, and implement."

Barriers identified were evident in participant responses, "this policy is relevant to my patient population, more clinicians should be educated," "make them more readily accessible, and have a website that lists all the hospital specific protocols," and "I wish the guidelines were all readily available in a binder or a paper folder." Because electronic resources are the "source of truth" for policy or guidelines at this health system, suggestions to provide paper binders and folders may undermine the availability of electronic sources.

Environmental Factors

Environmental factors such as organizational culture, infrastructure, social norms, and resources had significant influence on use of guidelines. Several advanced practice providers suggested the most important factor influencing the use of the local guideline was the recommendation by opinion leaders. Respected peers were trusted to judge the evidence, "the neurointensivist helped create the guideline," "endorsement by the physician," "senior staff/attending physicians recommend," "I was informed by a colleague," or "learned from the pharmacist." Proactive leadership had an impact on guideline use "my manager expects me to use the guideline," "it's hospital policy," and "much importance is placed on practice guidelines in this organization" were more frequently cited as reasons to use guidelines than not. Use of embedded links in the electronic health record to clinical decision support tools such as Up to Date, Clinical

Pharmacology, Epocrates, Access Medicine, Micromedex, Clinical Doc, PubMed, American Heart Association guidelines, hospital-specific guidelines, and standard order sets confirmed infrastructure support providing easy access to evidence.

Barriers in the learning culture at the clinical site were noted. When asked how participants were educated on the hospital specific guidelines, replies included, "no education, I read the policy myself," "on the job education," "a memo," and "I found them by overhearing a conversation." Other participants were "given a paper copy to read" or identified an inability to find guidelines on the health system website. Answers revealed a perception of inadequate orientation and ongoing education for the neuroscience advanced practice providers in relation to the hospital-specific clinical practice guideline.

Cognitive Factors

Cognitive factors including experience, competency, conceptual understanding, and self-efficacy swayed participants to use guidelines. Responses to specific knowledge questions about anticoagulation reversal in intracranial hemorrhage patients revealed expertise, knowledge, and strict adherence to protocol recommendations: "I refer to the health system website, follow the anticoagulation guideline protocol, discuss recommendations with attending staff and confer with pharmacy team" or "I stop aspirin and Plavix, assess PT/PTT/INR, CBC and administer platelet transfusions per protocol." Most responses to the clinical case studies revealed high level critical thinking with verbatim referral to the hospital guidelines. Specific recommendations for holding anticoagulant medications, reversal agent medication names and dosage recommendations, diagnostic laboratory tests with time frames, and blood pressure parameters were outlined in patient treatment plans. Many responses revealed an expert level of understanding. When a lack of knowledge was present, participants used guidelines to supplement their knowledge: "there are many new anticoagulant reversal agents, I know how to reverse antiplatelet agents, and it's the others that are more complex necessitating use of the guidelines."

Survey participants identified a lack of awareness as a barrier: "some emergency room physicians and advanced practice providers are not aware of the guidelines. They continue to give fresh frozen plasma (FFP) instead of prothrombin complex concentrates (PCC); they don't know or follow the guideline." Although one-half of respondents (53%) identified the top barrier as "impossible to keep up with all clinical practice guidelines in the field," "lack of knowledge or failure to have the guideline memorized," and "I did not know the guideline exists," most clinicians felt they were "familiar with guidelines in their field": "guidelines were readily accessible" (88%) and "practical to use" (88%).

Relationship of Results to Aims/Objectives

The purpose of this project was to seek understanding of what factors promote or prevent the implementation of evidence-based clinical practice guidelines at the point of care delivery. Perceptions of external and internal factors that influence the use of clinical practice guidelines in a population of neuroscience advanced practice providers were evaluated. The results from the survey add to the understanding of how clinical practice guidelines were used in a community hospital setting by a group of neuroscience nurse practitioners and physician assistants. The survey demonstrated a consistent use of the hospital-specific anticoagulation reversal protocol in the survey population. Minimal treatment variability was noted in qualitative responses to case scenarios. The use of evidence-based guidelines was an important step in translating knowledge into practice for this group of clinicians. Participants in the project were knowledgeable of, understood, and used guidelines to assist in clinical decision making with the ultimate goal of keeping patients safe and improving patient outcomes.

Impact of Results on Practice

The survey revealed that most respondents perceived clinical practice guidelines as valid tools to improve patient outcomes. Few of the failure modes anticipated by the prospective risk assessment process were realized. Use of evidence was improved by easily accessible, high-quality, well-developed local guidelines pertinent to the patient population served.

Despite the lack of a standardized process for educating clinicians to the hospital-specific guidelines, the majority of providers exhibited familiarity and a competent level of knowledge in the use of the hospital-specific guidelines in the patient scenarios. Through narrative responses for challenging patient scenarios, respondents exhibited proficiency in synthesis and integration of a complex set of guidelines to guide clinical decisions and treatment plans. Participants demonstrated appropriate use of the local anticoagulation reversal guideline content and most provided correct answers for the clinical case scenarios. If unable to provide answers, respondents stated that they would actively seek and consult a peer to obtain the correct information before proceeding with treatment. The survey highlighted the importance of using champions of change, such as respected colleagues, to engage clinicians in efforts to improve practice and adherence to standards. Findings from the survey were used to develop implications for practice.

Strengths and Limitations of the Project

No studies have examined the perceptions of neuroscience advanced practice providers in the use of clinical practice guidelines. This project sheds new light on the dynamic workflow of a clinician's use of clinical practice guidelines embedded in an electronic health record. One of the strengths realized by the project was an increased awareness of the hospital-specific anticoagulation reversal guideline. The survey served as an educational tool, encouraging respondents to review the guideline and discuss with peers before responding to case studies.

The increased attention of the project and survey may have led to a temporarily inflated response to the use of local guidelines resulting in a Hawthorne effect. Clinicians may have studied the hospital specific guidelines to answer the survey to perform well and "pass the test." The study is limited by a small sample size and the convenience sample of neuroscience advanced practice providers. Because the health system has multiple sites with multiple advanced practice providers, the sample may not be representative of advanced practice providers in the organization. Because of the small sample size, findings cannot be generalized to the advanced practice provider population at large.

Future Implications for Practice

A multifaceted approach is necessary to facilitate the use of clinical practice guidelines to improve patient care. Based on survey findings of barriers in the use of clinical practice guidelines, the following implications for practice are recommended:

1. Improve recognition and awareness of the current state.
2. Address ongoing education and competency.
3. Attain endorsement from administration.
4. Use a team approach with strong clinical leadership to address deficiencies.

The first step in the process is to evaluate the use of local clinical practice guidelines and assess barriers to use. Distribution of a confidential self-assessment survey to the intended users to identify obstacles, such as level of knowledge, attributes of the guidelines, or the context of practice are a method to increase advanced practice provider awareness and identify areas for process improvement.

Increased use of clinical decision support tools moves clinical practice guidelines more rapidly to the patient encounter. Education and training during orientation must include available electronic resources, access to and expectations of use of local guidelines appropriate to the service line. Survey results should serve as a needs assessment to identify high-risk, low incidence guidelines that require reinforcement during yearly ongoing competency assessment. Discussion forums during rounds or formal health system conferences should be encouraged to improve compliance to clinical practice guideline expectations.

Organizations must adopt a vision that embraces evidence-based practice, leadership support, and a focus on teamwork and collaboration. Identification of clinical champions from all members of the health care team to develop and implement local guidelines may improve the consistency of behavior. The entire multiprofessional team (physicians, advanced practice providers, nurses, and pharmacists) have a responsibility to participate in the development of best practices and a local standard of care. Health system–wide guideline development task forces may confer a "seal of approval" to promote trustworthy clinical practice guidelines. Commitment and endorsement need to come not only from clinical leadership, but administration as well. Because improving patient outcomes was a high correlate in the use of guidelines, development of a mechanism of audit and feedback specific to pertinent guidelines is necessary to encourage advanced practice providers to monitor neuroscience patient outcomes. Development of a quality scorecard based on performance would not only reinforce the learning culture, but allow the neuroscience team to assess and adjust performance to improve care processes and ultimately neuroscience patient outcomes.

Translating evidence efficiently to benefit patients in the daily demands of practice environments is fundamental to quality practice. As members of the patient care delivery team, advanced practice providers possess the expertise required to bring clinical practice guidelines to the bedside more quickly to improve the health, quality and safety of neuroscience patients.

ACKNOWLEDGMENTS

The author gratefully acknowledges the support and guidance of S.D. Krau, PhD, CNE Associate Professor, School of Nursing, Vanderbilt University and C. Thomson-Smith, MSN, RN, JD, FAANP, Assistant Dean Faculty Practice & Assistant Professor, School of Nursing, Vanderbilt University.

REFERENCES

1. Field MJ, Lohr KN, editors. Clinical practice guidelines: directions for a new program, Institute of Medicine. Washington, DC: National Academy Press; 1990.
2. Abrahamson KA, Fox RL, Doebbeling BN. Facilitators and barriers to clinical practice guideline use among nurses. Am J Nurs 2012;112(7):26–35.
3. Alanen S, Välimäki M, Kaila M, ECCE Study Group. Nurses' experiences of guideline implementation: a focus group study. J Clin Nurs 2009;18:2613–21.
4. Ebben R, Vloet L, Mintjes-de Groot J, et al. Factors influencing adherence to an emergency department national protocol. Eur J Emerg Med 2012;19(1):53–6.

5. Ebben R, Vloet L, Verhofstad M, et al. Adherence to guidelines and protocols in the prehospital and emergency care setting: a systematic review. Scand J Trauma Rescue Emerg Med 2013;21(9):1–16.

6. Legal Dictionary. Standard of Care definition. 2014. Available at: http://legal-dictionary.thefreedictionary.com/standard+of+care. Accessed December 28, 2014.

7. Buppert C. Nurse practitioner's business practice and legal Guide. 4th edition. Sudbury (MA): Jones & Bartlett Publishers; 2012.

8. Balas EA, Boren SA. Managing clinical knowledge for health care improvement. In: Bemmel J, McCray AT, editors. Yearbook of medical informatics 2000: patient-centered systems. Stuttgart (Germany): Schattauer Verlagsgesellschaft mbH; 2000. p. 65–70.

9. Laing L. The gap between evidence and practice. Health Aff (Millwood) 2007; 26(2):w119–21.

10. Flaherty ML. Anti-coagulant associated intracerebral hemorrhage. Semin Neurol 2010;30(5):565–72.

11. Moussouttas M. Challenges and controversies in the medical management of primary and antithrombotic-related intracerebral hemorrhage. Ther Adv Neurol Disord 2012;5(1):43–56.

12. Cervera A, Amaro S, Chamorro A. Oral anticoagulant-associated intracerebral hemorrhage. J Neurol 2012;259(2):212–24.

13. Aguilar MI, Hart RG, Kase CS, et al. Treatment of warfarin-associated intracerebral hemorrhage: literature review and expert opinion. Mayo Clin Proc 2007; 82(1):82–92.

14. McDermott RE, Mikulak RJ, Beauregard MR. The basics of FMEA. Portland (OR): Resources Engineering; 1996.

15. American Hospital Association, Health Research & Educational Trust, & Institute for Safe Medication Practices. Pathways for Medication Safety: Looking Collectively at Risk. 2002. Available at: http://www.ismp.org/tools/pathwaysection2.pdf. Accessed December 20, 2012.

16. National Research Council. Clinical practice guidelines we can trust. Washington, DC: The National Academies Press; 2011.

17. Greenhalgh T, Robert G, Bate P, et al. Diffusion of innovations in health service organisations: a systematic literature review. Malden (MA): Blackwell Publishing Ltd; 2005.

18. Brokel JM. Infusing clinical decision support interventions into electronic health records. Urol Nurs 2009;29(5):345–52.

19. Jao CS, Hier DB. Clinical decision support systems: an effective pathway to reduce medical errors and improve patient safety, decision support systems. Croatia (Europe): InTech; 2010.

20. NCCPA. Competencies for the physician assistant profession. 2012. Available at: http://www.nccpa.net/App/PDFs/Definition%20of%20PA%20Competencies%203.5%20 for%20Publication.pdf. Accessed December 29, 2013.

21. NONPF. Nurse practitioner core competencies. Washington, DC: NONPF; 2012.

22. Wong JM, Bader AM, Laws ER, et al. Patterns in neurosurgical adverse events and proposed strategies for reduction. Neurosurg Focus 2012;33(5):E1–8.

23. Council of State Neurologic Societies. Practice guidelines from the AANS/CNS joint guidelines committee. 2013. Available at: http://csnsonline.org/guidelines.php. Accessed December 28, 2013.

24. American Association of Neuroscience Nurses. AANN clinical practice guideline series. 2013. Available at: http://www.aann.org/pubs/content/guidelines.html. Accessed December 28, 2013.
25. Gaddis GM, Greenwald P, Huckson S. Toward improved implementation of evidence-based clinical algorithms: clinical practice guidelines, clinical decision rules, and clinical pathways. Acad Emerg Med 2007;14(11):1015–22.
26. Godin G, Bélanger-Gravel A, Eccles M, et al. Healthcare professionals' intentions and behaviours: A systematic review of studies based on social cognitive theories. Implement Sci 2008;3:36.
27. Bandura A. A social cognitive theory of personality. In: Pervin L, John O, editors. Handbook of personality. 2nd edition. New York: Guilford Publications; 1999. p. 154–96.
28. Nevid JS. Psychology: concepts and applications. 3rd edition. Boston (MA): Houghton Mifflin Company; 2009.
29. Cabana MD, Rand CS, Powe NR, et al. Why don't physicians follow clinical practice guidelines? A framework for Improvement. JAMA 1999;282(15):1458–65.
30. Larson E. A tool to assess barrier to adherence to hand hygiene guideline. Am J Infect Control 2004;32(1):48–51.

Simulation and Rubrics

Technology and Grading Student Performance in Nurse Anesthesia Education

Maria Overstreet, PhD, RN[a],*, Lewis McCarver, DNP, CRNA[b],
John Shields, DNP, CRNA[b], Jordan Patterson, BA[b]

KEYWORDS

- Simulation evaluation • Rubrics • Graded performance • Performance behaviors
- Nurse anesthesia • CRNA

KEY POINTS

- Observations of instructors can be subjective. Because of this subjectivity, it is imperative to provide clear and consistent information to learners.
- Objectives are the point of origin of clarity. Educators use objectives to define for learners what the primary focus will be in the classroom lectures or learning activities.
- Rubrics are tools to assist both learners and instructors with performance evaluations. A rubric is a tool used to assist scoring behaviors by defining criteria for evaluation and proficiency levels.
- To better define learner expectations, grading rubrics should reflect learner objectives provided to participants before their simulation experiences. A well-constructed rubric can provide a grading system to reflect learner performance for specific content in simulation exercises.

Videos of hand-off and initial assessment (Video 1); recruitment of the surgeon, hemodynamic manipulation, and fluid administration; communication and hypotension (Video 2) after declamping; provider collaboration and handover (Video 3); conclusion of the scenario and debriefing (Video 4) accompany this article at http://www.nursing.theclinics.com/

INTRODUCTION

Advances in technology have introduced many changes to nursing education, practice, and service. The use of simulation technology has introduced a challenge for simulation

---

Disclosures: None.
[a] Middle Tennessee School of Anesthesia, Vanderbilt School of Nursing, 315 Hospital Drive, Madison, TN 37116, USA; [b] Middle Tennessee School of Anesthesia, 315 Hospital Drive, Madison, TN 37116, USA
* Corresponding author.
E-mail address: m.overstreet@mtsa.edu

nurse educators: evaluation of student performance. Historically, student performance was evaluated in the classroom with written examinations and in the clinical setting by faculty or preceptor subjective observations. The subjectivity of student performance evaluation has been in need of improvement, both for learners and instructors.

Define Subjective

Subjective: "relating to the way a person experiences things in his or her own mind: based on feelings or opinions rather than facts."[1]

Because of the subjectivity of observations, it is imperative to provide clear and consistent information to learners. This clarity and consistency provides the nurturing support and transparency that learners need for a welcoming and warm teaching/ learning relationship. Objectives are the point of origin of clarity. Krau and Maxwell[2] (2011) identify educational objectives as a first step in the teaching process as well as guiding the educational and evaluative process. Educators use objectives to define for learners what the primary focus will be in the classroom lectures or learning activities. Simulation shares the same use of objectives. Simulation activities in a laboratory should begin with clear objectives shared between the learners and instructors. The learners should have information to support their simulation learning activities and know the expectations of their participation and performance.

Krau and Maxwell[2] describe how clear objectives are foundational to the development of an evaluation tool to measure learning. Because performance in a simulation activity may be single skill, multiple skills, or include attitude or application of a complex concept, clear objectives are foundational in the process of creating clear and consistent messages from instructors to learners.

DIFFERENCES IN ASSESSMENT AND EVALUATION

A simplistic method of discerning the difference in assessment and evaluation is to understand the purpose of the activity.[2] In performing an assessment, people gather data, analyze or interpret the data, and then form a direction or plan of action for the learner. The instructor gathers information to assess where the learner is at that time and makes a plan of how to assist in moving the learner forward. For an evaluation, the instructor is more focused on the final outcomes of an activity or performance. For example, an evaluation offers data about the extent to which criteria were met by the learner. Evaluations typically occur in either a formative or summative fashion, meaning the time at which the evaluation occurs (formative means during the educational process and intended to foster development of skill; summative means at the end of an educational offering and intended to judge stated goals).

In simulation, assessment and evaluation can occur in an almost simultaneous, or at least a continuous, fashion.

Tools such as checklists historically have been used to facilitate assessment/evaluation measures of learner performance. Rubrics have now become more popular with educators in providing increased direction and clarity for learners as well as instructors.

CREATING RUBRICS

A rubric is a tool used to assist scoring behaviors by defining criteria for evaluation and proficiency levels. Lasater[3] found that rubrics in simulation facilitate communication and provide a language that learners and instructors can use to aid feedback and discussion. Lasater[3] also found that rubrics assist in setting standards for learners to work toward. These findings reflect the thoughts of Krau and Maxwell[2] about defining clarity of performance expectation between learners and instructors.

The rubrics we have created identify the knowledge, skill, and attitude of the learner in discerning the various levels of performance criteria (**Fig. 1**). In our journey to using rubrics, we began with simple checklists that were turned into more complex checklists (**Tables 1** and **2**, respectively). We then were able to make the leap to rubrics for grading learner performance in simulation (**Table 3**).

This article presents information on grading rubrics and more specifically information about the use of grading rubrics in simulation exercises with student registered nurse anesthetists (SRNAs). It discusses performance evaluation in health care simulation with specific emphasis on SRNAs, our move toward rubrics in simulation and what we discovered, consistency among raters, improved definition of expectations, reasonable grade for performance, and emergence of a theme for remediation. It also discusses the software platform we use for our rubrics: ExamSoft. In addition, it provides video of a performance of a simulation exercise, abdominal aortic aneurysm (AAA) repair, with an accompanying rubric template and discussion of the eventual graded performance rubric.

PERFORMANCE EVALUATION IN HEALTH CARE SIMULATION EDUCATION, WITH AN EMPHASIS ON NURSE ANESTHESIA

Issenberg and colleagues[4] (2005) described studies showing that intense and deliberate practice in a focused domain may enhance learner performance in the acquisition, demonstration, and maintenance of skills mastery. Use of computer-controlled human patient simulators (HPSs) can help provide such an environment: SRNAs, under faculty supervision, have the opportunity to experience intense, focused, and deliberate practice in selected anesthesia-related skills.

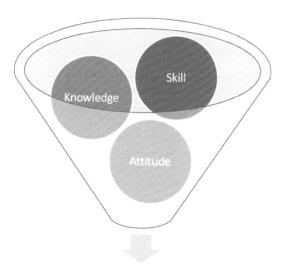

Performance criteria defined to provide clarity of expectations between learner and instructor

Fig. 1. Purpose of rubric in simulation exercises.

Table 1
Example of a simple checklist

Task to Perform	Done	Not Done
Communication with surgeon		
Call for assistance from second provider		
Phenylephrine bolus		
Ephedrine bolus		
Vasopressin bolus		
Calcium chloride bolus		
Epinephrine bolus		
Bicarbonate bolus		
Phenylephrine infusion titration		
Dopamine infusion titration		
Nitroglycerin infusion off		
Anesthetic agent titration		
Manipulate ventilator settings		
Trendelenburg position		
Normal saline/crystalloid bolus		
Albumin or Hespan/colloid bolus		
Red blood cell bolus		
Ask to reclamp		

This simple checklist outlines specific behaviors the learner must perform during the simulation. These behaviors do not describe all activities a learner must accomplish for the task to be considered done. With a simple (done/not done) checklist the level of performance and mastery of skill is not indicated.

Table 2
Example of an expanded checklist

Category	Points if Performed
Preparation of Work Site (3 points)	
Complete machine check	1
Complete equipment setup (laryngoscope, ETT, airway, suction on at head of table)	1
Complete medication check	1
Monitors (7 points)	
Apply pulse oximeter	1
Apply ECG leads	1
Apply NIBP	1
Obtain baseline vital signs *** (Critical step)	4

In this expanded checklist the learner is offered more information of specific actions to take during the simulation exercise and is given a weighted grade for specific categories which highlights the focus of the activity for a grade.

*** Indicates a critical step in the performance. If the critical step is omitted or not performed correctly, the learner will remediate and have an opportunity to perform again.

Abbreviations: ECG; electrocardiogram; ETT, endotracheal tube; NIBP, noninvasive blood pressure.

How Are Student Acquisition, Demonstration, and Maintenance of Skills Mastery Best Evaluated?

Evaluation of learner performance continually evolves. Our past HPS scenario debriefings guided learners in reflective practice and instructors provided formative assessments to students providing feedback specific to their individual strengths and weaknesses. Because the simulation exercises are part of an actual course, grades have been of concern. How can an activity be graded based on student performance with the overarching message that simulation exercises are a place to practice and fail while not harming any live patient? Historically, attendance and participation, not student performance, provided simulation course grades. Learners were responsible for attending and participating.

Although the use of computer-controlled human patient simulators in schools of nurse anesthesia is documented,[5–7] the use of grading rubrics for simulations with HPS scenarios in the academic education of SRNAs has not been described in nurse anesthesia literature. Use of summative assessments for students participating in HPS scenarios allows evaluation of specific competencies stressed in scenarios. We recognized that the ability to separate SRNAs who perform satisfactorily from those who do not for a given scenario at a specific time is vital, and may potentially be achieved through the use of grading rubrics. Rubrics for grading SRNAs in HPS scenarios offer a method to systematically measure learner performance. We have found that SRNAs showing critical thinking abilities and skills mastery in multiple simulation scenarios perform likewise in clinical practice.

MOVE TO RUBRICS IN SIMULATION
Greater Consistency Among Raters

Consistency from evaluators is unreasonable to expect without grading rubrics. A 5-minute to 10-minute HPS scenario for SRNAs offers numerous learner actions that may offer input into grade calculations. Rubric use for evaluation of SRNAs in meeting learner expectations focuses evaluator efforts and offers guides to assigning scores for different learner action categories. Without clear rubrics, areas of grading emphasis may lack focus; thus, the subjectivity of the evaluator can resurface. A learner should expect consistent grading among various instructors based on the categories and criteria presented in each rubric.

Rubrics Improve the Definition of Expectations to Learners

To better define learner expectations, grading rubrics should reflect the learner objectives provided to participants before their simulation experiences. Learner preparation before simulation experiences should mirror grading rubrics with learning objectives. The simulation scenario content should flow from the learning objectives and be reflected in the grading rubrics.[8] Three other areas to consider when developing a robust simulation exercise are to include for the learner evidence-based current practice patterns of nurse anesthetists, to address technical shortcomings of the human patient simulator,[9] and most importantly to appreciate various learner ability/performance levels. Well-defined rubrics should include all of the aforementioned content.

Rubrics can Provide Valid and Reasonable Grades for Performance

A well-constructed rubric can provide a grading system to reflect learner performance for specific content simulation exercises. Learner performance evaluations for each simulation exercise can then be incorporated into grading criteria for a course. Use

Table 3
Revised rubric for grading: abdominal aortic aneurysm (AAA)

Category		Scoring				
		4	3	2	1	0
Communication with surgeon	Notifies surgeon of: ○ Hypotension ○ Interventions ○ Exact blood pressure ○ Asks for assistance	Notifies surgeon of exact blood pressure, communicates treatment alternatives, updates surgeon on treatment provided and provides recommendations	Notifies surgeon of exact blood pressure, communicates treatment options and updates on treatment provided	Notifies surgeon of exact blood pressure when hypotensive	**Notifies surgeon of blood pressure decline**	Does not tell surgeon about hypotension
Management of hypovolemia	Reduces volatile agent Trendelenburg Administers colloid Administers crystalloid Administers blood	Administers blood, colloid, and crystalloid; provides Trendelenburg; reduces anesthesia gas	Administers blood, colloid and crystalloid; provides Trendelenburg	Transfuses blood and colloid in response to hypovolemia	**Transfuses blood or crystalloid only**	Does not transfuse any additional volume
Management of medications	Phenylephrine Ephedrine Vasopressin Calcium Bicarbonate Phenylephrine drip Dopamine drip Epinephrine	Administers at least 5 different medications in response to hypotension	Administers at least 4 different medications	Administers 3 medications	**Administers 2 medications**	Administers only 1 medication in response to hypotension

Safety	Drugs organized PPE Sterility Sharps	Drugs maintained in organized fashion, PPE used, handles sharps correctly while maintaining sterility	**Drugs maintained in organized fashion, PPE used**	Does not maintain drugs in organized fashion, PPE used	Does not maintain drugs in organized fashion, handle sharps correctly; medication error; no PPE —
Professionalism	Stands erect Eye contact Clear communication Direct interactions Respectful interactions	Stands straight and uses eye contact; communication is clear; interactions are honest; and others are treated with respect	**Stands straight and uses eye contact; communication is clear**	Stands straight and uses eye contact	Does not conduct self in a professional manner —
Communication effectiveness and handover	Effective communication Repeats specific order if appropriate Asks for clarification if unclear Not hesitant to ask for assistance Uses SBAR during handover	Repeats a specific order and asks for clarification if unclear; asks for assistance if needed; uses SBAR guidelines to receive/transfer a patient	**Repeats a specific order and asks for clarification if unclear**	**Repeats a specific order and asks for clarification if unclear**	Communication ineffective and does not ask for assistance —
Total points					

Bolded entries are crucial steps in the induction process and, if these steps are omitted or not performed correctly, the student will remediate and have an opportunity to perform again.

If a student does not receive a score equal to or greater than 80%, the student will remediate and have an opportunity to perform again.

A second failure after remediation may be grounds for dismissal from the program.

Abbreviations: PPE, protective personal equipment; SBAR, Situation, Background, Assessment and Recommendation.

of multiple simulation exercises and evaluators may reduce inconsistencies in evaluations.[10] We have discovered in our limited experience of using rubrics with simulation exercises that the rubric should be developed in conjunction with the simulation scenario so that the instructor can test the rubric as the simulation is tested for content and consistency among users.

Grading Performance May Identify Need to Remediate

Although satisfactory grades for a simulation experience do not guarantee satisfactory clinical performance, low grades for a scenario or simulation course may identify learners who could benefit from remediation opportunities. We have developed a remediation simulation program for those learners who need additional time, experience, or confidence. Each learner is given the opportunity to come back to re-perform a simulation exercise should they or their instructor request. Although the learner may not acquire the optimal score, remediation has proved to be an effective alternative to failure. Learners need a time to practice and to be graded. In our simulation program we have tried to incorporate both practice and performance. Learners are responsible at the outset for completing learning activities before simulation exercises (readings, videos, quizzes, and checklist/rubrics), responsible for their performance in the simulation exercise, and responsible for providing reflective insight on their performance during the debriefing immediately following the exercise. The instructor is responsible for clarity of expectations, objectives, grading, providing valuable expert feedback, and creating an environment supportive of learning.

RUBRICS USED TO FACILITATE STUDENT REGISTERED NURSE ANESTHETIST PERFORMANCE IN SIMULATION

Paired with didactic and clinical learning, simulation is an important aspect of nurse anesthesia education. Skills checklists and problem-solving outcomes historically were used to capture student abilities and comprehension during simulation. Evaluation was inconsistent, if not ineffective, because of variability in assessment by multiple instructors. In addition, performance expectations and desired behaviors were poorly defined and subject to interpretation. We have found that an effective evaluation tool, such as a rubric, can enhance the learning experience, provide a framework for the objectives, and minimize the subjectivity of the instructor.

PLATFORM USED TO CREATE RUBRICS

We decided as a team to use the rubric section of ExamSoft to create robust rubrics. In ExamSoft rubrics can be created and graded (**Fig. 2**). A feature that ExamSoft provides is the ability to share rubrics. This sharing feature allows uniformity of all rubrics for all instructors. Another feature ExamSoft offers is called tagging. In rubrics, categories created can be linked, or tagged, to specific learner outcome criteria. This tagging feature allows reporting on learner progress throughout simulations.

FIRST RUBRIC CREATED FOR GRADING STUDENT REGISTERED NURSE ANESTHETIST SIMULATION PERFORMANCE

We initiated a pilot study to create our first grading rubric for the SRNA simulation performance. We used 3 dimensions and 3 performance levels (**Fig. 3**). For the ExamSoft AAA rubric first attempt, dimensions were inserted as rows and described the 3 learning objectives (**Box 1**) associated with the simulation. The learning categories incorporated the Council on Accreditation for Nurse Anesthesia learning objectives

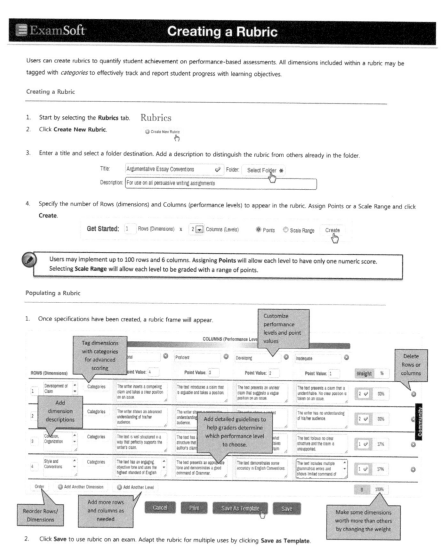

Fig. 2. Creating a rubric in ExamSoft: quick reference guide. (*Courtesy of* ExamSoft: quick reference guide; with permission from Examsoft Worldwide, Inc.)

and associated these in each dimension. Performance levels were tiered and based on performance of tasks during the simulation that were used in problem solving. Knowledge to perform these problem-solving tasks could be acquired by the learner from assigned readings before the simulation exercise and learners were prompted during the simulation with cues to performance. In preparation for the simulation, the student was provided with objectives (see **Box 1**) and a concise but thorough reading about the simulation-based anesthetic along with SRNA strategies (Appendix 1) to use to treat hypotension with volume replacement and multimodal pharmacology.[11–14] The 3 target behaviors for the AAA simulation were effective communication with the surgeon, effective management of hypovolemia using volume

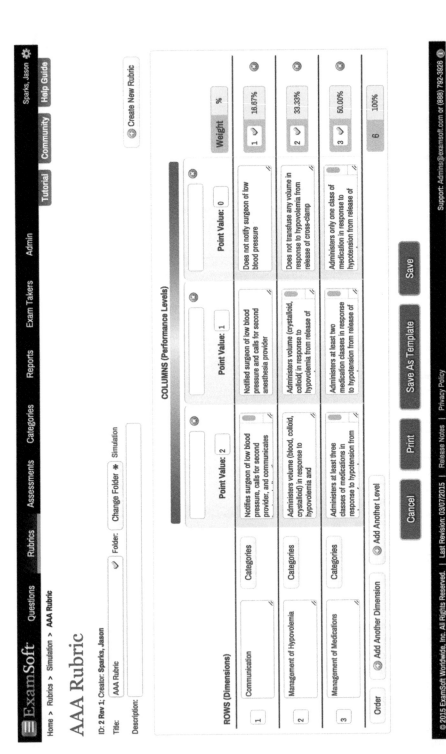

Fig. 3. ExamSoft AAA rubric first attempt. (*Courtesy of* ExamSoft: quick reference guide; with permission from ExamSoft Worldwide, Inc.)

Box 1
Objectives for vascular anesthesia: AAA repair simulation exercise

Objectives. The learner will perform the following behaviors appropriately during the simulation exercise:

1. Demonstrate adequate communication with surgeon during shock associated with aortic cross-clamp removal

2. Demonstrate appropriate use of volume resuscitation in treatment of acute hypovolemia associated with aortic cross-clamp removal–related shock

3. Demonstrate advanced use of multiple vasopressors and medications in treating hypotension associated with aortic cross-clamp removal–related shock

---

replacement, and multimodal use of vasoactive drugs in treating hypotension. Initially scoring was weighted heavily for one of the 3 tasks or target behaviors (pharmacologic treatment of hypotension).

LESSONS LEARNED IN THE MOMENT

While gathering data for evaluation of the rubric several issues immediately arose that required modification of both the rubric and learner preparation.

- The rubric was not readily available to the student as it was being piloted and changes may be made based on performance and grading.
- Learner performance varied in managing the hypotension, such that effective evaluation required expansion of the performance levels from 3 to 5 levels.
- During debriefing, the rubric was used to provide a scientific basis for performance evaluation, and immediate feedback revealed the rubric needed better structure and template of performance expectations.

The modified rubric was subsequently made available for the learner to review in preparation for the simulation. Because of the high fidelity (ie, realism) of the simulation, it offered the opportunity to evaluate other dimensions of learner behavior, including professionalism, safety behaviors, and handover between providers. The rubric was modified to include these additional dimensions (6 in total), with 5 performance levels instead of 3 (see **Table 3**).

ABDOMINAL AORTIC ANEURYSM RUBRIC DEVELOPMENT AND PERFORMANCE EVALUATIONS: ACCOMPANIED BY VIDEO

In the accompanying videos, the simulation exercise experienced by the student was to provide patient anesthesia for repair of an AAA. Anesthesia considerations, learner behaviors, and expectations were provided before the simulation in the form of a publication and grading rubric. After receiving handover the student was allowed to assess the patient's hemodynamics, vasopressor infusions, drug availability, and anesthesia level. Declamping of the aorta after the repair and subsequent hypotension were managed first by recruiting the surgeon through effective communication of hemodynamic status and potential interventions. Hypovolemia from blood loss and declamping were managed by infusion of blood, blood products, and crystalloids based on laboratory results and cardiac filling pressures. In addition to treating blood pressure with fluid resuscitation, vasopressors were administered along with treatment of acidosis. At the conclusion of the 10-minute simulation, handover and transition of care were returned to the learner. Debriefing followed the rubric and the objectives

Table 4
Rubric for grading: AAA learner performance via video link (● indicates student performed activity) student passed 96%

Category	Scoring				
	4	3	2	1	0
Communication with surgeon Notifies surgeon of: ● Hypotension ● Interventions ● Exact blood pressure ● Asks for assistance	Notifies surgeon of exact blood pressure, communicates treatment alternatives, updates surgeon on treatment provided, and provides recommendations	Notifies surgeon of exact blood pressure, communicates treatment options and updates on treatment provided	Notifies surgeon of exact blood pressure when hypotensive	**Notifies surgeon of blood pressure decline**	Does not tell surgeon about hypotension
Management of hypovolemia ● Reduces volatile agent ● Trendelenburg ● Administers colloid ● Administers crystalloid ● Administers blood	Administers blood, colloid and crystalloid; provides Trendelenburg; reduces anesthesia gas	Administers blood, colloid, and crystalloid; provides Trendelenburg	Transfuses blood and colloid in response to hypovolemia	**Transfuses blood or crystalloid only**	Does not transfuse any additional volume
Management of medications ● Phenylephrine ● Ephedrine Vasopressin Calcium Bicarbonate ● Phenylephrine drip Dopamine drip Epinephrine	Administers at least 5 different medications in response to hypotension	Administers at least 4 different medications	Administers 3 medications	**Administers 2 medications**	Administers only 1 medication in response to hypotension

Criterion	Items				
Safety	● Drugs organized ● PPE ● Sterility ● Sharps	Drugs maintained in organized fashion, PPE used, handles sharps correctly while maintaining sterility	**Drugs maintained in organized fashion, PPE used**	Does not maintain drugs in organized fashion, PPE used	Does not maintain drugs in organized fashion, handle sharps correctly; medication error; no PPE	—
Professionalism	● Stands erect ● Eye contact ● Clear communication ● Direct interactions ● Respectful interactions	Stands straight and uses eye contact; communication is clear; interactions are honest; and others are treated with respect	**Stands straight and uses eye contact; communication is clear**	Stands straight and uses eye contact	Does not conduct self in a professional manner	—
Communication effectiveness and handover	● Effective communication ● Repeats specific order if appropriate ● Asks for clarification if unclear ● Not hesitant to ask for assistance ● Uses SBAR during handover	Repeats a specific order and asks for clarification if unclear; asks for assistance if needed; uses SBAR guidelines to receive/transfer a patient	**Repeats a specific order and asks for clarification if unclear**	Repeats a specific order and asks for clarification if unclear; asks for assistance if needed	Communication ineffective and does not ask for assistance	—
Total points		20	3			23 out of 24 (96%)

Bolded entries are crucial steps in the induction process and, if these steps are omitted or not performed correctly, the student will remediate and have an opportunity to perform again.

If a student does not receive a score equal to or greater than 80%, the student will remediate and have an opportunity to perform again.

A second failure after remediation may be grounds for dismissal from the program.

Notes of instructor following review of video performance: learner performance graded start scenario 3:08; unclamp at 6:00; end 13:20; debrief until 18:50. Performed handover and assessment at beginning. Performed communication and management of hypotension 2 hours and 30 minutes into simulation. Provided effective collaboration and handover with second provider 6 hours and 45 minutes into simulation. Self-identified multiple areas of strengths and areas to improve during debriefing.

for the simulation and included effective communication, appropriate volume resuscitation, and effective use of vasopressors. Critiques of behaviors and rationale were referenced to the reading and rubric and focused on evidence-based practice.

GRADING OF LEARNER PERFORMANCE OF ABDOMINAL AORTIC ANEURYSM SIMULATION EXERCISE

In grading this simulation performance, the rubric was strictly followed and scoring was directed by learner actions associated with the level of performance. Hand-off and initial assessment (Video 1) by the student included behaviors from each of the dimensions and included recruitment of the surgeon, hemodynamic manipulation, and fluid administration. Communication and hypotension (Video 2) ensued after declamping, as the hemodynamic status was communicated and fluid bolus and vasopressor medications were administered. All 5 desired behaviors were performed by the student in the hypovolemia dimension, and were communicated to the surgeon. Four of the behaviors were performed in the management of medication dimension, including vasopressor drugs and treatment of acidosis with sodium bicarbonate. Second provider collaboration and handover (Video 3) presented an opportunity for the student to explore other interventions and rationale in a clinical context. Handover was detailed and followed the situation, background, assessment, and recommendation (SBAR) protocol, and the student's professionalism and interactions were of very high quality. Conclusion of the scenario and debriefing (Video 4) was inclusive during the handover to the second provider, and offered the opportunity for the student to be more interactive. Combined with a formal debrief at the conclusion of the scenario, the learner had outstandingly met the objectives of this simulation (**Table 4**).

SUMMARY

The use of simulation technology has introduced a challenge for simulation nurse educators: evaluation of student performance. Because of the subjectivity of observations, it is imperative to provide clear and consistent information to learners. This clarity and consistency provides the nurturing support and transparency that learners needs for a welcoming and warm teaching/learning relationship. A rubric is a tool used to assist scoring behaviors by defining criteria for evaluation and proficiency levels. Lasater[3] found that rubrics in simulation facilitate communication and provide a language that learners and instructors can use to aid feedback and discussion.

Although the use of computer-controlled human patient simulators in schools of nurse anesthesia is documented,[5–7] the use of grading rubrics for simulations with HPS scenarios in the academic education of SRNAs has not been described in nurse anesthesia literature. Creation of rubrics to replace checklists to evaluate learner performance is a team task. Multiple iterations of the rubric revealed more precise language and descriptions of expected learner behavior. This clarity assists learners in anticipation of activities as well as performance of activities. The clarity provided by the rubric assists instructors in providing valuable immediate and postactivity feedback and consistency among instructors (inter-rater reliability). During debriefing, the rubric was used to provide a scientific basis for performance evaluation, and immediate feedback revealed the need for better structuring and templating of performance expectations. Learner performances continue to improve and learners have begun to expect a higher level of transparency and clarity with acknowledgment of expectations.

Future steps include transitioning the simulation grading rubrics to clinical practice grading rubrics in an effort to offer more clarity to clinical preceptors, certified registered nurse anesthetists, and learners (student registered nurse anesthetists).

Translation of these behaviors from HPSs to live patient situations will take multiple iterations to discover similarities and exceptions that must be considered. Input from learners, instructors, and preceptors must drive this next initiative to be successful.

Please see the following links for more information.

Useful Web links:

How to write objectives

http://www.naacls.org/docs/announcement/writing-objectives.pdf

http://fitnyc.edu/files/pdfs/CET_TL_BloomsTaxonomy.pdf

Creating rubrics

http://rubistar.4teachers.org/index.php

Sample rubric

http://www.sites4teachers.com/links/redirect.php?url=http://www.congresslink.org/rubric.pdf

Oral presentation rubric

http://www.sites4teachers.com/links/redirect.php?url=http://www.louisianavoices.org/pdfs/Unit3/Lesson1/RubricForOralPresentation.pdf

Five best rubric tools

http://elearningindustry.com/the-5-best-free-rubric-making-tools-for-teachers

Sample rubric

http://steinhardt.nyu.edu/scmsAdmin/media/users/sa1636/MELZI_Grading_Rubric.pdf

file:///C:/Users/simdir/Downloads/Metler_Designing_scoring_rubrics_for_your_classroom.pdf

http://academic.pgcc.edu/~wpeirce/MCCCTR/Designingrubricsassessingthinking.html

---

SUPPLEMENTARY DATA

Supplementary data related to this article can be found online at http://dx.doi.org/10.1016/j.cnur.2015.03.001.

REFERENCES

1. Subjective. Available at: http://www.merriam-webster.com/dictionary/subjective. Accessed March 12, 2014.
2. Krau S, Maxwell C. Creating a tool to evaluate patient performance. Nurs Clin North Am 2011;46:351–65.
3. Lasater K. Clinical judgment development: using simulation to create an assessment rubric. J Nurs Educ 2007;46(11):496–503.
4. Issenberg SB, McGaghie WC, Petrusa ER, et al. Features and uses of high-fidelity medical simulations that lead to effective learning: a BEME systemic review. Med Teach 2005;27(1):10–8.
5. Fletcher J. AANA Journal course: update for nurse anesthetists – anesthesia simulation: a tool for learning and research. AANA J 1995;63:61–7.
6. Henrichs B, Rule A, Grady M, et al. Nurse anesthesia student's perceptions of the anesthesia patient simulator: a qualitative study. AANA J 2002;70(3):219–25.
7. O'Donnell J, Fletcher J, Dixon B, et al. Planning and implementing an anesthesia crisis management course for student nurse anesthetists. CRNA 1998;9(2):50–8.
8. Epstein RM, Hundert EM. Defining and assessing professional competence. JAMA 2002;287:226–35.

9. Schuwirth LW, van der Vleuten CP. The use of clinical simulations in assessment. Med Educ 2003;37(Suppl 1):65–71.
10. Boulet J. Summative assessment in medicine: the promise of simulation for high-stakes evaluation. Acad Emerg Med 2008;15:1017–24.
11. Miller RD, editor. Anesthesia, vol. 2, 6th edition. Philadelphia: Elsevier/Churchill Livingstone; 2005. p. 3376.
12. Roizen MF, Fleisher LA. Essence of anesthesia practice. 2nd edition. Philadelphia: W.B. Saunders; 2002. p. 377.
13. Mehta M, Taggert J, Darling RC, et al. Establishing a protocol for endovascular treatment of ruptured abdominal aortic aneurysm: outcomes of a prospective analysis. J Vasc Surg 2006;44(1):1–8.
14. Cheung AT, Pochettino A, McGarvey ML, et al. Strategies to manage paraplegia risk after endovascular stent repair of descending thoracic aortic aneurysms. Ann Thorac Surg 2005;80(4):1280–8.

APPENDIX 1: STUDENT REGISTERED NURSE ANESTHETIST STRATEGIES DURING THE ABDOMINAL AORTIC ANEURYSM REPAIR SIMULATION EXERCISE.

Perioperative risks

- Dependant on patient condition: high incidence of comorbid disease (hypertension, conorary artery disease, carotid disease, atherosclerosis of major vessels).

- Perioperative mortality of infrarenal aneurysms from the national database is 5.6% to 8.4% with the mortality of ruptured AAAs over the last 4 decades remaining at 50%. If all ruptured AAAs, including patients who died before reaching the hospital, were included the mortality could be greater than 90%.

- Nonlethal myocardial infarction 4% to 15%.

- Respiratory complications, 5% to 10%.

- Renal insufficiency, 2% to 5% (infrarenal), 17% (suprarenal).

- Bowel complications (intestinal ischemia).

- Paraplegia. Anterior spinal syndrome: loss of motor and pinprick sensation but preservation of vibration and proprioception. The patient has increased risk of neurologic complication if the aorta is clamped above the major anterior segmental medullary artery (artery of Adamkiewicz), which has variable origins: T5 to T8, 15%; T9 to T12, 60%; L1 to L2, 25%.

Perioperative considerations

- Preoperative: appropriate laboratory tests drawn, assess comorbidities, consider postoperative pain control (epidural vs intravenous [IV] patient-controlled anesthesia [PCA]), cell saver and cerebrospinal fluid (CSF) drain (discussed later), type and cross

- Monitoring. Invasive monitoring: arterial line, central line (central venous pressure [CVP] ± pulmonary artery catheter [PAC]); ± transesophageal echocardiography; ± CSF drain; neuromonitoring (MEPs [Motor evoked potentials]/SSEPs [somatosensory evoked potentials])

Operating room (OR) checklist
Emergent AAA

- Room warmed
- OR flat bed in room (for fluoroscopy)
- C-arm notified (check with OR nurse)

- Belmont and level I, primed
- Colloid (albumin plus Hextend)
- Consider cell saver
- Double/triple transducer connected
- Surgeons will access femoral artery for aortic balloon occlusion if combined interventional radiology procedure
- For interventional: do not induce anesthesia until aorta is occluded by the balloon, if possible

Access

- Arterial line: preinduction if possible
- Large-bore IV access: multiple (connected to Belmont and level I)
- Central line: can be placed later unless peripheral access not adequate

Elective AAA

- Arterial line
- Central line
- Large-bore IV lines
- Epidural: traumatic/bloody tap of epidural or CSF drain may require cancellation of procedure
- CSF drain: placed in high-risk patients for treatment/prevention of spinal cord ischemia
  - Redo-AAA/extensive aortic repair
  - Involves thoracic aorta
  - If combined stent procedure

Medications

Similar to medications for cardiac setup: heart box, fast-track box, syringes (nitroglycerine, 20 µg/mL; epinephrine, 10 µg/mL; phenylephrine, 100 µg/mL; ephedrine, 5–10 mg/mL). First-tier infusions: epinephrine, fenoldopam, nicardipine. Second-tier infusions: nitroglycerin, dopamine, vasopressin. Mannitol (12.5–25 g), heparin (50–100 units/kg), before cross-clamp on surgeon's request.

Infusions

- Normal saline carrier, stopcock manifold
- Fenoldopam (keep low dose [0.01–0.1 µg/kg/min] for renal perfusion; more data needed)
- Nicardipine: 1 to 4 µg/kg/min
- Epinephrine: start 0.01 µg/kg/min
- Vasopressin: start 0.04 units/min

Intraoperative

- Before cross-clamp
  - Consider renal protection: mannitol, loop diuretic, and dopamine are widely given despite studies showing little or no benefit. Fenoldopam infusion (a selective dopamine type 1 agonist) may be beneficial in dilating renal and splanchnic vasculature but more data are needed.
  - Heparin needs to be available 5 minutes before aortic cross-clamping; check activated clotting time (ACT) baseline, 3 minutes after heparin given and every 30 minutes thereafter while cross-clamped.

- During/after cross-clamp
  - Cross-clamp: sudden increase in afterload. Decrease afterload with vasoactive drugs (fenoldopam, nicardipine) to decrease Left ventricular wall tension. However, maintain a CVP greater than 10 mm Hg.
  - However, when aneurysm is opened, back-bleeding may lead to sudden hypovolemia (maintain CVP, get ready for bleeding).
  - Organs distal from clamp will be hypoperfused and ischemic; turn off lower body warmer.
- Infrarenal. This avoids most major organs and has the least hemodynamic effect and fewest postclamp complications. Patients still have decreased renal blood flow and increased renal resistance, and therefore renal protection should be considered.
- Suprarenal. Renal, spinal, and lower extremity ischemia are possible.
- Supraceliac. Hemodynamic changes can be drastic and likely require dilators to decrease afterload. The kidneys, intestines, and liver are ischemic and thus coagulopathy, acidosis, and renal dysfunction are likely.
  - Need arterial blood gases every 10 minutes during clamp
  - Fraction of inspired oxygen (FiO_2) 100%
  - Correct acidosis (Sodium Bicarbonate)
  - Stabilize electrolytes
  - Volume, calcium, and consider sodium bicarbonate before clamp release
  - Keep CVP more than 15 mm Hg before clamp release
  - Have pressors ready and in line during unclamping
  - Coagulations, thromboelastography, complete blood count after clamp release
- After clamp. Response to unclamping depends on clamp time and location of clamp. It is important to communicate during unclamping with surgery to optimize cardiac output. During unclamping, large hemodynamic swings can occur and vasoactive medications need to be readily available. Partial or complete reclamping may be needed to optimize hemodynamic state if the patient does not tolerate initial unclamping.

Postoperative considerations

- Blood pressure and heart rate control
- Extubation depends on OR course and fluid shifts/presser requirements
- Analgesia: IVPCA versus epidural
- Neurologic deficit (see earlier discussion of CSF drains)

OR AAA summary checklist

Preoperative: consent, history and physical, laboratory tests, epidural, CSF drain, awake arterial line, large peripheral IV

OR: room warm, OR flatbed, Belmont/level 1 wet down, double transducer (arterial line, central line), central line set up (ultrasonography, gown, gloves), arterial line set up, IV set up

Drugs: induction drugs, cardiac box, mannitol, heparin, syringes (epinephrine, phenylephrine, ephedrine, nitroglycerin, esmolol)

Drips on stopcock manifold: normal saline carrier, epinephrine, vasopressin, fenoldopam, nicardipine

Induction: hemodynamically stable

Intraoperative:

Before cross-clamp. Start fenoldopam/dopamine, consider mannitol, Lasix, dopamine for renal protection. Check baseline ACT before giving heparin 5 minutes before cross-clamp. Recheck ACT 3 minutes after giving heparin and then every 30 minutes.

During cross-clamp. Determine cross-clamp level. If supraceliac, the kidneys, intestines and liver will be ischemic and coagulopathy, acidosis, and renal dysfunction likely: check arterial blood gases every 10 minutes, FiO_2 100%, correct acidosis (Sodium Bicarbonate), stable electrolytes, keep CVP approximately 15 mm Hg, maintain pressure.

If CSF drain in place. Initial goal 10 to 12 mm Hg, zero at atrium, if SSEP/MEPs decrease. Drain 10 mL (no more than 20 mL/h), optimize blood pressure.

After clamp. depends on clamp location; have drips ready and treat blood pressure aggressively with fluid/pressors.

Geriatric Simulation

Practicing Management and Leadership in Care of the Older Adult

Sally Miller, MS, RN[a],*, Maria Overstreet, PhD, RN[a,b]

KEYWORDS

- Geriatric • Simulation • Nursing • Leadership • Management

KEY POINTS

- Nurse educators are currently challenged to prepare nursing students with the knowledge, skills, and attitudes necessary to provide care to a vastly growing population of older adults.
- Multiple factors contributed to the creation of a nursing clinical simulation (NCS) focused on the care of the older adult, including increased nursing student enrollment making appropriate student clinical placement sites more difficult to obtain, a deficit of nurse faculty specializing in geriatrics, and an increase in hospitalized older adults.
- The geriatric management and leadership NCS was created by faculty with expertise in simulation, debriefing, and geriatric nursing.
- Nurse practitioner students may be added to the NCS to portray the role of health care provider and can serve as a valuable collaborative effort between various educational levels of students.

Nurse educators are currently challenged to prepare nursing students with the knowledge, skills, and attitudes necessary to provide care to a vastly growing population of older adults. According to the Centers for Disease Control and Prevention,[1] patients age 65 and older accounted for 43% of hospital days. Therefore, there is a great likelihood that nursing students will be assigned to provide care for older adult patients during acute hospital clinical experiences. Hospitalized older adults have multiple complex needs, including comorbidities, sensory deficits, and polypharmacy.[2] The complexity of providing nursing care for an older adult provides nursing students with opportunities to assess, prioritize, intervene, and advocate for the older adult and family, as well as experience being a member of an interdisciplinary health

Disclosures: None.
[a] Clinical Learning Center, Vanderbilt University School of Nursing, Godchaux Hall 316, 461 21st Avenue South, Nashville, TN 37240, USA; [b] Center for Clinical Simulation, Middle Tennessee School of Anesthesia, 315 Hospital Drive, Madison, TN 37115, USA
* Corresponding author.
E-mail address: sally.m.miller@vanderbilt.edu

http://dx.doi.org/10.1016/j.cnur.2015.03.008
0029-6465/15/$ – see front matter © 2015 Elsevier Inc. All rights reserved.
nursing.theclinics.com

care team. The American Association of Colleges of Nursing (AACN)[3] explicitly states that students must have opportunities to learn about and practice management and leadership principles. AACN-Hartford[4] previously called for nursing students to become involved in simulation and laboratory activities involving this special population.

Multiple factors contributed to the creation of a nursing clinical simulation (NCS) focused on the care of the older adult, including increased nursing student enrollment making appropriate student clinical placement sites more difficult to obtain, a deficit of nurse faculty specializing in geriatrics, and an increase in hospitalized older adults. With these factors in mind, NCS became a resource tool for the creation of a clinically relevant experience for nursing students to practice management and leadership in the care of the older adult. NCS can augment or even replace clinical practice hours by providing specific learning opportunities that may not occur during nursing students' clinical time to provide real patient care.[5]

This article describes the geriatric management and leadership NCS experienced by nursing students during a four year period. It begins with a brief background of simulation and geriatric care. Content and application of the NCS are described, including tables with detailed information necessary for other educators to implement this NCS. Next, lessons learned are explored. Finally, recommendations for future educational opportunities are proposed.

BACKGROUND OF GERIATRIC MANAGEMENT AND LEADERSHIP NURSING CLINICAL SIMULATION

Simulation, still in its infancy and becoming increasingly utilized in nursing education, is documented to promote teamwork, provide practice crisis resource management, and assist in the understanding of roles and responsibilities, decision-making, and communication.[6] Scant research exists on the use of NCS in assisting nursing students to learn the necessary skills of management and leadership in the clinical setting. Guhde[7] and Reed and colleagues[8] describe NCSs with a focus on leadership and management. A simulation was designed for students to experience various roles such as nurse, nursing assistant, and family member. Students valued the use of critical thinking skills and increased awareness of the importance of patient assessment. However, it was Guhde[7] who recognized the value of NCS debriefing in which students gained skills in communication, prioritization, clinical decision-making, leadership, and clinical judgment.

Reed and colleagues[8] described an NCS in which students were asked to manage an 8-bed unit with medical-surgical patients. The students and faculty engaged in multiple roles. They reported that the faculty was able to identify when students made good clinical decisions within the context of a complex environment. The NCSs by Reed and colleagues[8] and Guhde[7] provided nursing students an opportunity to practice leadership and management skills. However, neither group had an NCS focused on the specialized needs of providing care of older adults.

On the other hand, Bamber and colleagues[9] described the use of NCS as a final learning event following an unfolding case study spanning 4 semesters. This NCS includes intensive care of the older adult as well as end-of-life care. Paquette and colleagues[10] used standardized patients to simulate an older adult with dementia, delirium, and heart failure. Nursing students had the opportunity to practice family support and education of the older adult. Both Bamber and colleagues[9] and Paquette and colleagues[10] focused simulated learning events on the older adult patient; however, leadership or management objectives were not specified.

GERIATRIC MANAGEMENT AND LEADERSHIP NURSING CLINICAL SIMULATION

The geriatric management and leadership NCS was created by faculty with expertise in simulation, debriefing, and geriatric nursing. Faculty with expertise in medical and surgical nursing, leadership, and management were asked to review content for accuracy and offer suggestions. This NCS was used to augment clinical hours for the final practicum of senior level baccalaureate students in an accelerated nursing program. Three hours were allocated for groups of 6 students to perform the NCS. Three hours allowed sufficient time for patient scenarios to evolve, time management situations to ensue, student practice, and repetition of skills, and debriefing.

Three objectives drove the content for the NCS: management, leadership, and care of older adults. Specific information from AACN[3] and AACN-Hartford[4] were used in the creation of objectives, patients, and scenarios. In addition to physical assessment and interventions, psychosocial issues such as caregiving, end-of-life decisions, care transitions, and autonomy were incorporated in the NCS.

Instructions or Rules

Instructions are discussed with students before the beginning of the simulation. The students are advised to perform skills accurately, treat the mannequins as they would treat real patients, and conduct themselves professionally as if in an authentic clinical setting. Although the students participating in the simulation have been previously oriented to the simulation environment, they receive reminders about what interventions can be performed on the mannequins (such as giving injections, running intravenous fluids, or changing dressings). To make the NCS more dynamic, faculty and staff members are recruited to participate in the simulation in various roles such as family and health care providers.

Creating a safe and trusting learning environment is an important aspect of simulation and allows students to practice, make mistakes, and correct their actions without harm to real patients.[11] To promote a safe learning environment, students are reminded their performance as well as that of their peers is to remain confidential.

Time and Structure

The NCS is divided into 3 sections. The first 30 minutes includes introductory remarks, rules and expectations, and discussion of objectives. Students are informed they will use knowledge acquired from didactic classes, skills practiced in laboratory and clinical experiences, and principles of management and leadership in the care older adult patients with medical-surgical diagnoses. The students listen to a prerecorded audio report from the night charge nurse as their first introduction to the patients. The pretaped report is a short summary of each patient, including physical status, vital signs, psychosocial issues, and pending laboratory work. Roles and work assignments are decided by the students.

During the second 90 minutes, students provide actual nursing care. They take vital signs, perform assessments, provide personal care, administer medications, and have the opportunity to make nursing judgments based on patient data collected or information received. Students refer to a note card with a brief, bulleted role description and responsibilities. For example, the charge nurse card includes: analyze workloads, make assignments, contact primary care providers, and transcribe orders. The staff nurse card includes instructions to perform focused physical assessments, administer medications, initiate and update plans of care, and delegate appropriate duties.

Students have access to simulated electronic health records and are expected to enter patient data in these charts. Included in the electronic health records are current orders, history, physical, medication administration records, nursing notes, intake and output records, vital signs, laboratory, and other miscellaneous reports. Internet access is available for students to retrieve policies, procedures, or medication reference information.

The students are informed that faculty or staff may enter the simulation and will wear a nametag to specify who they are and their role. For example, a nametag may read Kay Smith, Respiratory Therapist. Faculty and staff participants are encouraged to accomplish a single objective at a time and not to overact. For example, an actor enters the simulation as a family member and approaches the student with concerns about the newly prescribed diet and asks for clarification for home management. This engagement allows the student to practice time management skills, prioritization of care, and discharge teaching.

The final hour includes debriefing and rounding at the bedside. The debriefing is structured to occur immediately following the simulation experience. Students gather in an adjacent classroom and the 7 components of debriefing identified by Overstreet[12] are followed to facilitate students' reflection on the events of the NCS.

The student as charge nurse is asked to explore how she or he felt managing the other students as staff nurses. The other students are asked to offer the student charge nurse feedback on her performance. The team is asked if they would make any changes to the assignments based on what they now know about the patients. Nursing care specific to management of the older adult is discussed. The students in the staff nurse role are asked to discuss which of their 2 patients they assessed first and offer their rationale. For example, feedback is offered and discussion ensues for a student's appropriate decision to assess a patient with community-acquired pneumonia, preexisting dementia, and acute confusion before assessing a patient awaiting discharge. Students are asked to discuss the type of tasks they delegated and how they communicated their needs to the charge nurse or the resource nurse, and if or how they followed up on the delegation. The group then discusses their interactions and communication with health care providers and simulated family members.

Time is reserved at the end of the last hour to perform bedside rounding to explore any unanswered questions or issues. Students are asked to give a brief overview of each patient at the bedside. This time is valuable in soliciting student comprehension of the older patient's specific care needs through discussion of promoting and retaining functional ability, recognition of acute confusion, restraint reduction, and prevention of hospital-acquired complications. Students are asked to describe how their patient's aging process and comorbidities affect the admitting diagnosis. Bedside rounding provided the opportunity to address any misperceptions about common age-related changes versus diseases and pathologic conditions.

Application of learning from the simulation environment to real patient care was accomplished by asking students what they learned in simulation that they would take to their next clinical day. Students voiced an increased awareness of factors affecting prioritization of care, how to work as a team, the need to gather all data before contacting health care providers, and increased confidence communicating with health care providers. The students also overwhelmingly thought the NCS prepared them for increased independence with clinical decision-making at the point of care.

Patients

Case studies of patients typically found in an older adult medical-surgical population portray common and recurring admission diagnoses and conditions. Examples of simulated admission diagnoses include patients with a fractured hip, knee replacement, near-syncopal episode, and community-acquired pneumonia (**Table 1**). These patient scenarios incorporate patient safety issues such as prevention of catheter-associated urinary tract infections, fall reduction, and pressure ulcer prevention.

Events

To make the simulation dynamic and realistic and offer students practice responding to commonly occurring clinical issues, situations are introduced in a variety of ways. Cue cards placed on the medium-fidelity mannequins alert students to patient requests such as the need for pain medication or the onset of nausea (**Table 2**). Live vocals streamed to the high-fidelity mannequins increases realism and encourages interaction between the student and the patient. Notes taped on the mannequins signify conditions such as pedal edema or pressure ulcer formation and are meant to be discovered during the student's physical assessment. Faculty and staff are recruited to portray family or interdisciplinary team members. To increase the realism of the simulation, persons not known by the students are invited to participate. Phone calls from the control room into the simulated unit allow students to practice professional communication such as identifying themselves professionally, requesting passwords before giving patient status information, and receiving and repeating laboratory results or orders. These interpolated situations create opportunities for students to prioritize, manage time, delegate tasks, or communicate with the charge nurse or other health care team members during performance of their duties (see **Table 2**).

An example of a situation for students to practice communication, maintain confidentiality, advocate for the patient, educate family, and perform a nursing task is outlined next. A faculty member acting as a patient's daughter calls into the simulation unit and asks to speak with the nurse caring for her father. In keeping with the objective of professional communication, students practice identifying themselves professionally when answering the phone and asking the caller for the patient-specific password. The actor provides the password and insists the urinary catheter scheduled to be removed should not be taken out because her father had difficulty urinating after his last surgery. This conversation allows the student to practice professional communication, promote patient confidentiality, listen to the family member's concern, educate family members regarding the risk of urinary tract infection, maintain patient autonomy, remove the urinary catheter, and monitor the patient after catheter removal.

Other preplanned situations that students have an opportunity to respond to are built in to the simulation (see **Table 2**). For example, students must manage an elevated digoxin level, acute confusion superimposed on mild dementia, fluid overload, and pain management in advanced dementia. These patient problems provide students the opportunity to gather additional data, make clinical judgments, communicate with health care providers, receive orders, and take action.

Moulage

The mannequins are moulaged to portray older adults and props such as wigs, glasses, hearing aids, and other personal items are used (see **Table 1**). In addition, the mannequins are outfitted with equipment relevant to their chronic and acute diagnoses. For example, one mannequin has a first-day postoperative knee replacement with medical equipment, including an intravenous infusion, a drain affixed to his knee under a bandage, and an indwelling urinary catheter. Another mannequin portrays a patient with dementia and acute confusion and is seated in a bedside chair with her urinary catheter tubing wrapped in her hand. In addition to wigs and personal items,

Table 1
Patients in case study

Patient: Age, Gender Admitting Diagnosis Past Medical History	Moulage: All Mannequins had Gray, Black or Light-Colored Wigs	Simulator Settings
1 81, female Fractured left femur Hypertension, congestive heart failure, arthritis, macular degeneration, sickle cell anemia	Glasses Dressing on hip Primary intravenous with completed transfusion	BS: Crackles BP: 156/88 HR: 90/irregular RR: 20
2 80, male Pneumonia Chronic obstructive pulmonary disease, hypertension, coronary artery disease	Glasses Incentive spirometer Urinal Oxygen by nasal cannula Saline lock Antibiotic	BS: Wheezes BP: 140/90 HR: 88/regular RR: 18
3 80, male Right total knee replacement Arthritis, left knee replacement	Hearing aid Knee wrapped in elastic bandage with drain Urinary catheter Primary infusion	BS: Clear BP: 104/80 HR: 88/regular RR: 18
4 90, female Fractured right femur, fractured right ulna Anxiety disorder	Patient-controlled analgesia pump Splint on right wrist Leg supported by pillow Urinary catheter	BS: Clear BP: 98/56 HR: 90/regular RR: 10
5 86, male New-onset atrial fibrillation Syncope	Glasses Telemetry box Orthostatic blood pressure results indicated by 3 × 5 card on mannequin's arm Saline lock	BS: Clear BP: 98/60 HR: 99/irregular RR: 20

#	Patient	Findings	Vitals
6	80, female Rapid atrial fibrillation Dementia, hypertension, diabetes, anemia, gout, chronic constipation, herpes zoster	Hijab (Muslim head covering) Stage 1 pressure ulcer on coccyx, dressing on lateral malleolus	BS: Coarse crackles BP: 94/70 HR: 88/regular RR: 20
7	80, female Community-acquired pneumonia Dementia	Glasses on bedside table Up in chair Urinary catheter Saline lock	BS: Coarse crackles BP: 140/90 HR: 88/regular RR: 18
8	81, male Laser transurethral resection of prostate	Urinal with pink-tinged urine and small clots	BS: Clear BP: 138/78 HR: 89/regular RR: 16
9	85, female Fractured femur, contact isolation Postoperative admission	Femur dressing Oxygen by mask Oxygen saturation 88% Urinary catheter with scant output Infusion 150 mL/h	BS: Crackles BP: 158/90 HR: 110, premature ventricular complexes RR: 22
10	86, male Dementia, aspiration pneumonia Dementia, new admission, do-not-resuscitate order	Gastric feeding tube	BS: Coarse crackles BP: 130/80 HR: 98/regular RR: 24, continuous moaning

Abbreviations: BP, blood pressure; BS, breath sounds; HR, heart rate; RR, respiratory rate.

Table 2
Essential events and actors

Patient	Situation Description	Actors (Faculty, Staff, or Visitors)	Desired Action by Student	Geriatric Goal Management or Leadership Emphasis
1	Bedside visit script: "Can you tell me what diet, activity, and medications she'll need when she comes home?"	Family member	Engages family in discharge teaching	Functional status, nutrition, polypharmacy Communication, discharge planning
2	Cue card on mannequin: Wet voice and frequent clearing of throat after taking morning medications	No actor	Elevate head of bed, check oxygen saturation, encourage to cough, notify provider, remove food and fluids	Nutrition or hydration, safety Communication, prioritization, report change of status
3	Telephone call script: "I don't want you to take the urinary catheter out. He had trouble urinating after his last surgery."	Family member	Decision whether to remove catheter per postoperative orders or to leave in per daughter's request	Autonomy, prevention of catheter-associated urinary tract infection Communication, confidentiality, time-management
4	Cue card on mannequin: Groggy, difficult to arouse, low respiratory rate	Preoperative anesthesia visit cues student to decreased respiratory rate. Or, student recognizes low respiratory rate provides intervention and calls Rapid Response team	Recognizes low respiratory rate, stops pain medication, calls Rapid Response team or provider	Drug dosing and clearance Prioritization, reporting change in status, uses SBAR
5	Telephone call script: "This is the laboratory calling with a critical digoxin level."	Faculty	Student does not administer medication until morning laboratory result obtained, contacts provider	Drug dosing and clearance Communication, prioritization, time-management

6	Cue card on mannequin: Patient grimacing, writhing and moaning	No actor	Reports to provider information obtained about family's decision for "Do Not Resuscitate"	Palliative and end-of-life care, pain assessment and treatment, prevention of pressure ulcers Interdisciplinary team communication
7	Cue card on mannequin: "I need to go to the bank..." or bedside visit script: "Mom seems really confused today."	Family member	Recognizes and reports acute confusion and change from baseline	Acute confusion in patient with dementia, safety Communication, delegation, prioritization
8	Cue card on mannequin: "I feel shaky and I'm really hungry."	No actor	Recognize diabetic status, check blood glucose, give juice and notify health care provider	Interaction of chronic and acute conditions Communication, delegation, prioritization
9	Cue card on mannequin: "Help me! I can't breathe!"	No actor	Recognize fluid overload, stop IV, increase oxygen, call Rapid Response or provider, comfort patient	Interaction of chronic and acute conditions Communication, delegation, prioritization
10	Bedside visit script: "What's wrong with him? Help him!"	Family member	Elevate head of bed, call Rapid Response or Respiratory Care, provide support to family member	Ethical issues, advance directives, Communication, delegation, prioritization

Abbreviations: IV, intravenous; SBAR, Situation-Background-Assessment-Recommendation.

vital signs and breath sounds consistent with the simulated scenarios are programmed into the mannequins (see **Table 1**).

LESSONS LEARNED

This simulation has been conducted for 4 consecutive years and several revisions have occurred based on faculty observation, and faculty and student feedback. Revisions have included a brief discussion at the beginning of the simulation to prepare students for professional telephone communication on a hospital unit, a skill rarely practiced during the hospital clinical experiences. A universal health care template, Situation-Background-Assessment-Recommendation (SBAR), is used to provide consistency in reporting patient information to other health care providers. Students are encouraged to review leadership and management principles as well as geriatric coursework before the simulation. The ideal number of students to perform this NCS is 6 to 7. This number allows active participation of all students. Students perform the role of the graduate nurse, thus fostering their confidence in bedside decision making.

SUMMARY

Although this simulation was conducted for senior Bachelor of Science in Nursing students, the patient cases and scenarios are easily adaptable for various levels of students. The patient and faculty interactions can be made as simple or complex as desired, tailoring the NCS to the particular level of the student. Nurse practitioner students can be added to the NCS to portray the role of health care provider and can serve as a valuable collaborative effort between various educational levels of students. This template can be used by multiple specialties within and outside of nursing. This NCS can be transformed into a multidisciplinary team simulation. It creates a safe environment for students to learn other's roles and responsibilities as well as evidenced-based care of the older adult.

REFERENCES

1. Centers for Disease Control and Prevention. National hospital discharge survey: 2007 Summary 29. 2010. Available at: http://www.cdc.gov/nchs/nhds.htm. Accessed July 31, 2011.
2. Meiner SE. Gerontologic nursing. 4th edition. St. Louis (MO): Mosby; 2011.
3. American Association of Colleges of Nursing. The Essentials of Baccalaureate Education for Professional Nursing Practice. 2008. Available at: http://www.aacn.nche.edu/Education/pdf/BaccEssentials08.pdf. Accessed July 29, 2011.
4. American Association of Colleges of Nursing. Recommended Baccalaureate Competencies and Curricular Guidelines for the Nursing Care of Older Adults: A Supplement to The Essentials of Baccalaureate Education for Professional Nursing Practice. 2000. Available at: http://www.aacn.nche.edu/Education/pdf/AACN_Gerocompetencies.pdf. Accessed July 29, 2011.
5. Cato ML. Using simulation in nursing education. In: Jeffries PR, editor. Simulation in nursing education. New York: National League for Nursing; 2012. p. 1–10.
6. Gaba DM. Crisis resource management and teamwork training in anaesthesia. Br J Anaesth 2010;105(1):3–6.
7. Guhde J. Using online exercises and patient simulation to improve students' clinical decision-making. Nurs Educ Perspect 2010;31(6):387–9.
8. Che'Reed C, Lancaster RR, Musser DB. Nursing leadership and management simulation creating complexity. Clinical Simulation in Nursing 2009;5(1):e17–21.

9. Bamber M, Graven L, Abendroth M, et al. Embedding an unfolding geriatric case exemplar into nursing simulation. Clinical Simulation in Nursing 2010;6(3):e108.

10. Paquette M, Bull M, Wilson S, et al. A complex elder care simulation using improvisational actors. Nurse Educ 2010;35(6):254–8.

11. Rudolph JW, Simon R, Rivard P, et al. Debriefing with good judgment: combining rigorous feedback with genuine inquiry. Anesthesiol Clin 2007;25(2):361–76.

12. Overstreet M. Ee-chats: the seven components of nursing debriefing. J Contin Educ Nurs 2010;41(12):538–9.

The Influence of Technology in Nursing Education

Stephen D. Krau, PhD, RN, CNE

KEYWORDS

- Text mining • Data mining • Technology • Meaningful use • Telehealth • HIT
- Nursing education

KEY POINTS

- The complexity of the relationship between nursing and technology becomes greater with the advent of new technology and technological devices.
- Faculty who are in the clinical area on a limited basis, and for nurses who are not involved in decisions related to the adoption of technology, terms and concepts related to technology can be misconstrued or misunderstood.
- Some major terms used in reference to technology and technological approaches such as meaningful use, as well as data mining (DM), along with concepts related to telehealth can only enhance the intricate relationship between nursing and technology.
- Keeping current with new technologies and concepts that affect optimal patient outcomes is a mandate for all nurses as they work with the technology and guide patient education related to technology.

INTRODUCTION

There is much progress in the development of new technology and technologic modalities for either directly or indirectly improving patient care, as new innovations are created every day. There has been a great deal of discussion regarding how new technology has been seen as a hindrance to patient care by decreasing the time nurses spend in patient care, as well as regarding expenses that have emerged in purchasing programs and providing education and the rapid evolvement that literally makes yesterday's invention, obsolete today. Nurses have identified that technology also has the potential for depersonalization and objectification of patients. The potential for technology to affect patient individuality and subjectivity and create an alienation between the

Disclosure: None.
School of Nursing, Vanderbilt University Medical Center, 461 21st Avenue South, Nashville, TN 37240, USA
E-mail address: steve.krau@vanderbilt.edu

Nurs Clin N Am 50 (2015) 379–387
http://dx.doi.org/10.1016/j.cnur.2015.02.002
0029-6465/15/$ – see front matter © 2015 Elsevier Inc. All rights reserved.

patient and health care providers with their caring purpose is clear. The complexity of the relationship between technology and nursing care is not new.[1]

This complexity is further intensified by the new terms and concepts that continue to inch into the vocabulary and discussions; this is evident not only in nursing practice but also in the society as a whole. For example, who could have guessed a decade ago that there would be talks about "sexting," much less all of the legal and ethical issues that have ensued.[2] Understanding the various terms to describe technology in health care and conceptual terms related to health care is an ongoing task. For nurses who are not involved in technological decisions, and for faculty who have students in a clinical setting on a limited basis, the exposure to these concepts and terms can be restricted. Terms and concepts are heard in discussions, and in a nonsystematic context, can be misinterpreted or misunderstood. As part of an ongoing process, there are some basic terms and important concepts used in the arena of technology that should be understood by all nurses. There are many technology formats for education and learning, as well as simulation; the focus in this article is on technology seen in the clinical arena and research and often discussed by nurses. Students may overhear these words and come to the instructor for clarification. Nurses at the bedside may be unclear about what some of these concepts and terms actually entail. Understanding these terms and concepts is integral to the use and discussion of some of the many technological innovations.

When discussing technology, the focus could be on any one of a thousand concepts; the concepts explained in this article include terms related to health information technology (HIT) and meaningful use. Slipping from other technological areas are those terms that center on data management and data use such as text mining and DM. Monitoring devices and telehealth systems continue to carry some mystique for the novice nurse and nursing students. In addition, the recent importance of early warning systems (EWS) has emerged, because these systems provide a valuable tool for the early detection of deterioration in patient status, prompting quick intervention. Even when the names and concepts make sense in general, the meaning that these terms hold for nurses and nursing students can easily be misinterpreted or misunderstood.

Health Information Technology

The report from the Institute of Medicine on the future of nursing makes a recommendation that nurses be involved in the development of new approaches to technology such as HIT, to advance as well as to improve health care.[3] HIT systems are those that are based on technology and are used to access, exchange, automate, and enhance decision making; provide support to health care professionals as well as patients; and promote behaviors that enhance health and wellness.[4] As such, HIT has the potential to affect health and health care in a myriad of ways. For example, this impact can be focused on improving the quality and the cost of health care; it can also expand the range of health care. There is recent evidence that it can play a significant role in the management of disease processes.[5,6] HIT specifically refers to those technologies that permit health care professionals to improve outcomes by sharing and using information, gather information from electronic health records (EHRs), collaborate through sharing information via secure information networks, allow electronic prescribing, as well as engage patients and their families in care via technological methods.[4]

Meaningful Use

Although the term meaningful use carries a strong semblance to the suggestion of the term's connotation, the term has been operationalized to have specific considerations. This term is not a generic one as could be construed, but actually incorporates very specific parameters for what constitutes meaningful use. Passage of governmental reform and legislation including Health Information Technology for Economic and Clinical Health (HITECH), a component of the American Recovery and Reinvestment Act of 2009, Public Law11–5, and the Affordable Care Act has had a tremendous impact on the health care system in the United States.[7] HITECH created a program that provides financial incentives for eligible health care institutions to use electronic health care records (EHRs) in a fixed way. The law includes US $19.5 billion for incentives to health care agencies and health care professionals who use technology in a meaningful way, which is based on the development and use of EHRs.

As such, meaningful use does not imply that better health care results from adopting technology itself, but rather through the exchange and use of information to best affect the clinical decisions that occur at the point of care.[8] The Alliance for Nursing Informatics, which is composed of 25 organizations, issued a document stating that "Meaningful use of EHR systems should strive for nothing less than an integrated healthcare community that is patient centered and promotes usable, efficient, and seamless information flow."[9]

The meaningful use program is designed in 3 stages. The first stage, which took place from 2011 to 2012, was to focus on capturing data and sharing information. The second stage within a 2014 time frame was to focus on the use of technology to advance clinical processes. The third stage, which is going to occur in 2016, is focused on the use of meaningful use directed at improving outcomes.[10] In order to qualify for the governmental incentives, health care organizations and health care providers must demonstrate that they have met clear criteria for meaningful use.

The meaningful use criteria identifies standards to advance the use of HIT in health care. A summary of meaningful use standards specific to Medicare and Medicaid standards are identified in **Box 1**.

One of the issues identified with meaningful use and the use of electronic health care records (EHR) in general is that it might not be pervasive enough to assist patients and families in the participation, and ultimately, the success of its use. The meaningful use criteria does not emphasize patient involvement or patient perception enough for some health care providers who maintain that the success of use of EHRs is contingent on engaging patients and their families.[11] As nurses advocate for patients and their families, this omission can be perceived as a flaw in the operationalization of "meaningful use." While technologies considered in meaningful use, such as EHRs,

---

Box 1
Meaningful use standards operationalized by Medicare and Medicaid

1. Use certified electronic health care records to track, record, and exchange information.
   a. Use computerized physician order entries
   b. Record demographics and vital signs
   c. Maintain problem lists that are up to date
   d. Evaluate insurance eligibility and submit claims
   e. Exchange key clinical data
   f. Maintain privacy and security
2. Capture and submit specific clinical quality measures
3. Provide patients an electronic copy of their health information

directly involve patients and their families, they could also represent a platform for improving access to care, improving quality of care, empowering patients, and providing support between office visits. Some advocates think that meaningful use should include an assessment of the patient's experience as they engage with health care providers and institutions.[11]

Generating New Knowledge for Decision Making

With the expansion of EHRs and the overwhelming amount of information to which health care professionals have access, there are new modalities of harnessing this information. Through using this information and creating algorithms, and models, this information may yield additional information that is not known or not well understood. In essence, old information can be clarified, and even new knowledge can be created from these vast data systems. These processes can lead to knowledge that could be instrumental in clinical decision making and assuring optimal patient care.

Two terms that have come to the forefront related to obtaining and using knowledge from various data banks, including EHRs, are data mining and text mining.[12] Both involve accessing and extracting information from a large volume of documents. DM is the process in which useful knowledge and information is obtained from data banks. The goal of DM is to access information for further analysis and potential decision making.[12,13] Text mining is a more comprehensive process than DM in which there is mining of unknown and obscure parts of information from structured and semistructured text. Although very similar, there are elements of a priori algorithms and association rules that form a basis for text mining. These techniques are used for the enhancement of nursing diagnosis, improvement of consistency in the use of nursing terms, and reduction of time in the production of new ideas and concepts. DM is not just a single method or single technique but rather a spectrum of different approaches that search for patterns and relationships of data.[12] The methodological basis of DM is the discernment of patterns and relationships in large quantities of data that results in the construction of models that can help the assignment of class labels through the use of statistical methods, artificial intelligence to the management of databases.[14]

Both text mining and DM involve the use of a computer to access and organize data. Text mining is essentially the discovery of new or unknown information from large amounts of different unstructured textual resources. Extracted information is linked together to create new facts or ideas to be explored by more empirical means of investigation. When considering DM, patterns are discerned from natural language text as opposed to databases. Another aspect of text mining is related to web mining in which the input is unstructured and free text, whereas the web sources themselves are structured. The goal is to generate genuinely new information. This mining is different from simple information retrieval in which no genuinely new information is found. With information retrieval or what is commonly called a web search the health care professional is looking for something that has already been confirmed or validated.

The value of DM and text mining tools is in the application of these models in programs that analyze the vast amounts of information related to health care. When considering the tremendous data generated by patient health care visits, information in EHRs, medication errors, prescriptions, the filling of prescriptions, and specific physician notes, there is information that might be extrapolated into patterns that could improve patient outcomes and overall health care. There are many commercial text mining programs and tools, and there is much discussion about the efficacy and value of all these various programs. The importance of these processes becomes stronger with more frequent use and through the comprehension of health care providers who can connect these processes to their clinical practice.

Evidence

Although there are many studies that demonstrate the use and value of DM, the one of particular note is a study that applies it to improve the diagnosis of neonatal jaundice.[15] The investigators validated the usefulness of DM. In this study the researchers concluded that "the main finding of this study showed that DM techniques are important and valid approaches for prediction of neonatal hyperbilirubinemia."[15] The inference is that DM is useful to support medical decision making, and in this case contributes to improved diagnostics.

Daily Activity Monitors

With so much communication and so many devices able to convey information, and receive information, the implementation of daily activity monitors has modernized health promotion and disease management.[16,17] There are multiple devices available for monitoring daily activities, and some of them will affect the efficacy in practice. These devices vary in their usability, security, measurement parameters, support system, and convenience.

When exploring these devices, some of the mystique disappears when one considers pedometers that have been used for decades. The principle is similar, although current devices do much more than measure steps. Activity monitors can be used to measure multiple physiologic occurrences such as sleep cycle, calorie expenditure, heart rate, skin temperature, blood glucose levels, and activity classification.[17] These devices can also measure to what degree a goal was obtained in activity for a specific period.

Daily activity monitoring devices have been the focus of many companies. Some have been very successful, whereas others have fallen by the wayside. The evolution of activity monitoring devices continues. Although they are used more commonly today, and many associate their inaugural emergence with computers, activity monitoring devices in some form have been around since 1920.[17] Although not considered medical devices by the US Food and Drug Administration,[18] the use of monitoring devices and now apps has been flourishing since the mid-1960s (**Fig. 1**).

Daily activity monitoring devices are a mainstay in the health care system and allow the patient more self-care with regard to decision making based on information. Many devices have a variety of peripherals that can attach to phones, computers, tablets, and exercise machines. **Fig. 2** shows the Nike running watch, Basis watch, Jawbone UP with peripherals, and Fitbit One with peripherals. Although intimidating at first, many of these become as common as watches for many patients.

Nurse's knowledge of these devices and issues related to safety, privacy, and efficacy can only be obtained through thorough examination of the types of devices and the specific patient need. Depending on the health state of the patient, and the patient's specific needs, nurses are postured to help patients make decisions and to teach them about the different devices. It is now commonplace in some facilities to see patients bring their devices with them on admission. A more thorough discussion of the devices and types is warranted should frontline nurses or students be engaged in the decision-making process.

Evidence

At present, there is a lack of vigorous studies to support the value of the use of activity device to the consumer. The various companies that make these devices market them more based on the idea and the theoretically value that these devices may have for their customers. Most certainly this is partly because of the lack of involvement by the US Food and Drug Administration for approval. The next step in the evolution of

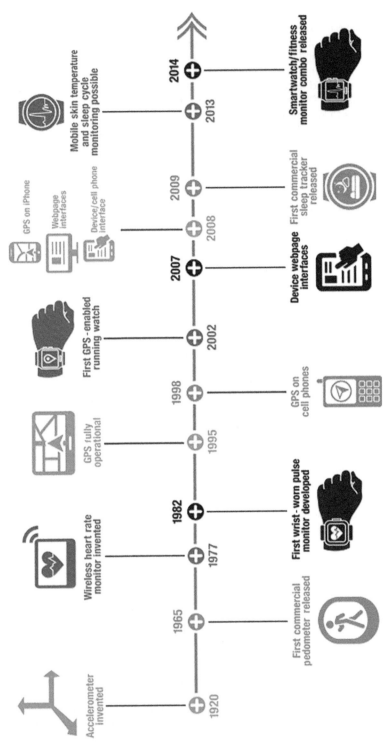

Fig. 1. The evolution of activity monitoring devices. (*From* Mancuso PJ, Thompson M, Tietze M, et al. Can patient use of daily activity monitors change nurse practitioner practice? J Nurse Pract 2014;10(10):789; with permission.)

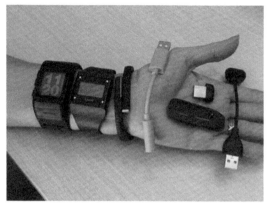

Fig. 2. Some devices with their peripherals. (*From* Mancuso PJ, Thompson M, Tietze M, et al. Can patient use of daily activity monitors change nurse practitioner practice? J Nurse Pract 2014;10(10):788; with permission.)

monitoring devices should include strong studies with large populations to determine the overall value of these devices.

Early Warning Scores Using the Electronic Medical Record

Along with providing vast amounts of data for mining, the health care record can also be used as a tool to assist the nurse in the detection of early patient status compromise in order to promote safety and enhance optimal patient outcomes.[19] There is often a subtle decline in patients' conditions 8 to 12 hours before an event, which can allow time for the health care team to identify patients at risk.[20]

Evidence

The use of EWS in conjunction with the electronic medical record and nurse alerts has been found to improve patient care and to enable early recognition of the need for emergent care. The use of the EWS has also been shown to assist in the education of nurses and in their personal development of autonomy and critical thinking skills.[20] The EWS can provide a guide for new nurses as they develop skills in determining a patient's overall condition, as well as recognizing even the most subtle changes in patient status. The EWS can also help nurses determine trends that might otherwise go unnoticed.

Telehealth

The Health Resources and Services Administration explains that telehealth is "the electronic information and telecommunications technologies to support long distance clinical health care, patient and professional health-related education, public health, and health administration."[21] Within the scope of nursing, one might hear this referred to as "telehealth nursing" and "telenursing".[21] At present, telehealth is not a nursing specialty area, but it is not hard to imagine that this technology will be needed in every nurse's skill set in the near future. Some of the devices and their uses are listed in **Table 1**.

Telehealth is being delivered in many inpatient and outpatient settings. Telehealth can provide such important services as telestroke, teledermatology, telepediatrics, teleneonatology, telepsychiatry, and telecardiology to many underserved areas.[22] The use of telehealth allows communication between patients and health care providers by improving access to care, regardless of the location (see **Fig. 2**).

Table 1
Some of the uses of telehealth technology

Remote monitoring devices	These devices allow patients to connect with health care professionals from their communities, or from their homes. Systems can include real-time connection such as videoconferencing. Some systems are asynchronous and allow the patient to answer such questions as "how is your heart rate this morning?" Replies are recorded and sent to the health care provider whose early detection of a potential problem can ameliorate exacerbation of the problem, and potentially a hospital visit
Remote physical assessment peripherals	These are similar to daily activity monitors; however, these allow patients to submit data from their home to the health care provider. These devices can include weight scales, pulse oximeters, glucose monitors, medication tracking equipment, and even "intelligent toilets." Data can be sent as real time, or can be stored and recorded to be sent later. These devices allow the tracking and display trends in patient information. In addition, some of these even allow for alerts should the heart rate become too high or a there be an extraordinary weight loss or gain
Mobile health (mHealth) devices	These are wearable sensors that can track information in real time. These devices can track and transmit information ranging from glucose levels to movement and balance
Personal health record apps	These apps are for mobile devices; they can hold patient information such as medication reminders and health history as well as collect environmental triggers for some respiratory issues, such as amount of pollen in the air or smog

Adapted from Grady J. Telehealth: a case study in disruptive innovation. Am J Nurs 2014;114(4):40; with permission.

SUMMARY

There are clearly implications for nursing education with advancement of this technology. Some suggest that technology might even be disruptive to the traditional ways in which nurses are taught, and that instead of passive learning, students should have the opportunities to apply and synthesize.[23] The newer generations of nursing students come with knowledge and skills related to much technology that they will use in nursing. It is instructors from previous generations who are the immigrants to the digital generation of nursing students and new nurses. However, it is essential that the terminology used in the description and understanding of new technologies be clear and understood by all nurses.

REFERENCES

1. Barnard A, Sandelowski M. Technology and humane nursing care: (ir)reconcilable or invented differences? J Adv Nurs 2001;34(3):367–75.
2. Mattey B, Diliberto GM. Sexting - it's in the dictionary. NASN Sch Nurse 2013; 28(2):94–8.
3. Institute of Medicine. The future of nursing: Leading change, advancing health. Report recommendations. Available at: http://www.iom.edu/~/media/Files/Report%20Files/2010/The-Future-of-Nursing/Future%20of%20Nursing%202010%20Report%20Brief.pdf. Accessed February 1, 2015.

4. HealthIT.gov. Health information technology. Health information technology site. Available at: http://www.healthit.gov. Accessed February 1, 2015.
5. Brammer RS, McKethan C, Buntin M. Health information technology: transforming chronic disease management and care transitions. Prim Care 2012;39:327–44.
6. Gauthier K. Starting the conversation: a health information technology tool to address pediatric obesity. J Nurse Pract 2014;10(10):813–9.
7. McQuade-Jones B, Murphy J, Novak T, et al. Nurse practitioners and meaningful use: transforming health care. J Nurse Pract 2014;10(10):763–70.
8. Martin KS, Monsen KA, Bowles KH. The Omaha system of meaningful use: applications for practice, education, and research. Comput Inform Nurs 2011;29(1):52–8.
9. Sensmeier J. Alliance for Nursing Informatics statement to the Robert Wood Johnson Foundation Initiative on the future of nursing: acute care focusing on the area of technology. Comput Inform Nurs 2010;28(1):63–7.
10. EHR incentives and certification. Available at: http://www.healthit.gov/providers-professionals/meaningful-use-definition-objectives. Accessed February 1, 2015.
11. Ralston JD, Coleman K, Reid R, et al. Patient experience should be part of meaningful use. Health Aff 2010;29(4):607–13.
12. Lao P, Chu W, Chu W. Evaluation of Techniques in constructing a traditional Chinese-language nursing recording system. Comput Inform Nurs 2014;32(5):223–31.
13. Goud R, Hasman A, Peak N. Development of a guideline-based decision support system with explanation facilities for outpatient therapy. Comput Methods Programs Biomed 2008;91(2):145–53.
14. Worachartcheewan A, Nantasenamat C, Isarankura-Na-Ayudhya C, et al. Identification of metabolic syndrome using decision tree analysis. Diabetes Res Clin Pract 2010;90(1):e15–8.
15. Duarte F, Abilio O, Freitas A. Applying data mining techniques to improve diagnosis in neonatal jaundice. BMC Med Inform Decis Mak 2012;12:143–8.
16. Topol E. The creative destruction of medicine: how the digital revolution will create better health care. New York: Basic Books; 2012.
17. Mancuso PJ, Thompson M, Tietze M, et al. Can patient use of daily activity monitors change nurse practitioner practice? J Nurse Pract 2014;10(10):787–93.
18. Lynch S. Silicon Valley Business Journal. Available at: http://www.bizjournals.com/sanjose/news/2013/09/23/fda-details-what-health-apps-it-plans.html. Accessed February 1, 2015.
19. Albert BL, Huesman L. Development of a modified early warning score using the electronic medical record. Dimens Crit Care Nurs 2011;30(5):283–92.
20. Whittington J, White R, Haig KM, et al. Using an automated risk assessment report to identify patients at risk for clinical deterioration. Jt Comm J Qual Patient Saf 2007;33:569–74.
21. Health Resources and Service Adminstration. Telehealth. n.d. Available at: http://www.hrsa.gov/ruralhealth/about/telehealth. Accessed February 1, 2015.
22. Henderson N, Tearsanee CD, Smith M, et al. Nurse practitioners in telehealth: bridging the gaps in healthcare delivery. J Nurse Pract 2014;10(10):845–55.
23. Grady J. Telehealth: a case study in disruptive innovation. Am J Nurs 2014;114(4):38–45.

Faculty Development in Simulation Education

Beth F. Hallmark, PhD, RN

KEYWORDS

• Technology • Simulation • Nursing • Faculty education

KEY POINTS

- Although there still remains much discussion on how to train faculty in simulation; the development of standards for faculty training and certifications for simulation educators is a positive move toward consistency.
- Much work remains to get nurse educators to a level of proficiency with simulation education.
- Many educators have not had formal training in how to use simulation. Many learn from others who may or may not have had formal education in simulation technology.

Health care educators typically begin their careers as professionals in the clinical area, without formal education courses in how to teach. Sometimes health care providers transition into education because of their desire to impact the future of health care. Over the past 10 years, education in nursing has changed and simulation is a new teaching technology being used. "Despite persistent or increasing pressure to use simulation, faculty remain inadequately trained and simulation remains under used."[1] Unfortunately, this lack of training of how to use simulation in education can translate into poor educational pedagogy. Nursing educators have traditionally been faculty from traditional nursing backgrounds with little experience in educational theory and training.[2] According to Poindexter,[3] "The role of a nurse educator is an intersection between nursing knowledge, values, and skills and teaching knowledge, values and skills." Training the nurse educator to effectively achieve this union is a subject that is not without controversy. Nursing faculty are first trained to be professionals that care for patients in some realm. Once a nurse decides to transition to the role of faculty the path taken to achieve this varies. In 2010, the Council on Collegiate Nursing Education published expectations for faculty preparation in bachelor of science in nursing programs. These recommendations outline the level of education of nursing or doctoral preparation expected by the academy and make specific recommendations for all doctoral programs: "should make available additional courses in

Disclosure Statement: None.

College of Health Sciences, Belmont University, 1900 Belmont Boulevard, Nashville, TN 37212, USA

E-mail address: beth.hallmark@belmont.edu

Nurs Clin N Am 50 (2015) 389–397

http://dx.doi.org/10.1016/j.cnur.2015.03.002

0029-6465/15/$ – see front matter © 2015 Elsevier Inc. All rights reserved.

nursing.theclinics.com

educational methods and pedagogies, and provide teaching experiences that include mentoring and supervision given the expectations for those graduates who will be involved in an academic role."[4]

A project funded by the Carnegie and The Atlantic Philanthropies (2010) examined how professionals are educated. This was a comparative study that took place over several years and examined three areas of nursing professional education: (1) how theory and scientific methodology is learned, (2) how skills are mastered, and (3) how nurses are taught professional identity.[5] Culminating from this project was a book, *Educating Nurses: A Call for Radical Transformation.*[5] Within this publication there are many recommendations related to nursing education. Of particular interest is the recommendation related to the preparation of nursing faculty to include teacher education courses in programs for master's and doctoral degrees. "Qualified and competent nurse educators facilitate the development of qualified and competent nurses prepared to assume successful nursing careers."[3]

The use of simulation as a teaching methodology within health care education is no different. Many educators have not had formal training in how to use simulation. Many learn from others who may or may not have had formal education in simulation technology. Because of their interest in technology they are placed in the role of simulation educator by default. This article introduces the importance of training educators and clinicians to use simulation technology according to defined standards and recommendations. A literature search revealed a dearth of research related to faculty training. I describe some programs in place across the United States that have been developed to facilitate education of faculty in use of simulation technology and methodology.

BACKGROUND

Healthcare in the United States was forever changed in 1999 when the Institute of Medicine published its report To Err is Human.[6] This report illuminated that as many as 100,000 people die every year in the United States as a result of preventable medical errors. This report dramatically increased public awareness of patient safety and medical errors. However, there is evidence that the report greatly underestimated the number of sentinel events and cost associated with medical errors. Today it is estimated that the cost of medical errors is $1 trillion and between 250,000 and 400,000 deaths annually.[7,8] In addition to medical errors that result in death or harm to patients, there has been an alarming shortage of nursing staff and faculty. Nursing education has been forced to explore ways to increase the number of nursing graduates and the pool of nurse educators. Historically nursing education has evolved into a profession that is well respected and considered rigorous in academic settings.

Clinical sites for the purpose of nursing students to practice are also scarce in many regions of the country, leading the administration of academic institutions and their practice partners to seek alternatives to inpatient clinical experiences.[9] The recent economic crisis has led to many nursing schools being left without adequate faculty and staff even in the midst of the well-documented nursing shortage. To address the increased incidences of medical errors and the resulting injury and/or death of patients, advocacy groups and accreditation bodies, such as The Joint Commission, National Quality Forum, and National Patient Safety Foundation, have all supported projects that improve patient safety and the education of nurses related to patient safety. Educating patients, and the staff that care for patients, must be purposeful and directed to address the errors and knowledge gap that exists. The overarching goal for multiple projects was to reduce harmful medical errors and keep the patient population safe and healthy. Nursing education cannot ignore this national cry for change in teaching methodologies.

Nursing faculty have responded to this national challenge by vigorously seeking new technology and cutting edge pedagogy. Simulation is one such pedagogy that provides for active learning methods that can afford students a "hands-on" experience that resembles actual clinical experiences. Clinical experiences include instruction in nursing education that consists of nursing students caring for live patients in real health care settings. The lack of available clinical sites, and the shortage of nursing faculty, has mandated alternatives to "practicing" on live patients. The ability to mimic lifelike situations in a laboratory setting using simulation has afforded nursing students with the opportunity to care for patients that they may never have the option to care for in the clinical area. Nurse educators have used simulation for decades. Early on, nurses injected water into an orange to simulate the skin of a real person. Nursing education has come a long way since those first rudimentary simulations.

Today's high-fidelity simulators provide the student the opportunity to perform invasive procedures, such as endotracheal intubation and chest tube insertion. Computerized technology allows the faculty to program these mannequins to mimic real patient situations and ultimately assess the student's ability to respond to changes in patient conditions at the point of care. Subsequent to the completion of the actual bedside simulation event the debriefing occurs. Training faculty to use this technology effectively and facilitate the debriefing is imperative to the successful integration of simulation pedagogy. Research in the area of high-fidelity simulation within nursing education is still in an infancy stage.

Simulation education is being integrated at an increased pace across the country. In 2014, the National Council of States Boards of Nursing released the results of a longitudinal multisite study that stated up to 50% of specific clinical experiences can be replaced using simulation.[10] "The Accreditation Council on Pharmacy Education (ACPE) has also approved the use of simulation in IPPEs for up to 20% or 60 hours of the total 300 hour experiential education requirement."[11] Other disciplines, such as physical therapy, occupational therapy, respiratory therapy, social work, and prehospital emergency medical technicians and paramedics are integrating simulation into their curricula. The increased focus of safety has called for more interprofessional education. Such programs as TeamSTEPPS have gained in popularity and often use simulation as a tool to train the trainers in interprofessional simulation.

THEORETIC SUPPORT FOR SIMULATION EDUCATION

Two prominent educational theories are used frequently to support simulation education: constructivism and active learning. "Constructivist theory suggests one has to experience the world to know it."[12] The constructivist believes the learner, through an active process, constructs the knowledge, taking into account what the learner already has experienced in life. The role of the faculty in the process of the "construction of knowledge" must be discovered. "A constructivist teacher is one who designs learning experiences that are active, where the learners are 'doing'; reflecting on and evaluating their learning experiences, and building on previous learning experiences to construct new knowledge and meaning."[12] Preparing faculty to use simulation as a constructivist teaching methodology fits well into the constructivist theory in that the learner engages in an active process and can incorporate their life experiences.

The American Association of Colleges of Nursing released in October of 2008 a revision of The Essentials of Baccalaureate Education for Professional Nursing Practice and, in agreement with the Association of American Colleges and Universities[13] position on Baccalaureate Education, clearly stated the strategies used for educating nurses must include "the widespread use of powerful, active, and collaborative instructional methods."[14] Active learning is best described as the students learning is active versus passive, hands-on and real-time involvement in the process. "Active learning involves providing opportunities for students to meaningfully talk and listen, write, read, and reflect on the content, ideas, issues, and concerns of an academic subject."[15]

Simulation exercises are active learning, hands-on, real-time opportunities where students can apply classroom knowledge and practice skills. How students best learn is defined by their learning style and their ability to think reflectively; combining the idea of how a teacher presents the material in terms of active or passive (hands-on or didactic, respectively) with how a student best learns. "New technologies provide opportunities for more realistic replications for teaching problem solving and clinical reasoning in nonthreatening environments."[16] High-fidelity simulation in health care was first seen in the area of anesthesia and the training of emergency medical personnel.[17] Simulation is a form of active learning in the truest sense, allowing students to make mistakes on simulated patient mannequins. This activity allows them to practice their skills while not having to fear the outcome of the potential for causing patient harm. According to Decker,[18] "instrumental to the learner's success" is a faculty member that has been trained with a particular set of skills.

THEORETIC SUPPORT FOR FACULTY TRAINING IN SIMULATION

In reviewing the current literature I found little evidence to support faculty training from a theoretic standpoint. Waxman and Telles[19] state "simulation trainers may be expert nurses in the clinical setting, yet they may be novices when learning to write and run scenarios using high fidelity simulations"; this supports the use of Benner's novice to expert theory when considering faculty training. Although several theories may be applicable to faculty training, the fact remains that most faculty are novices when they begin to use simulation as a tool to support student learning. Benner's novice to expert theory supports the need for well-developed education and intentional planning for faculty development in the use of new technologies, such as simulation.

BARRIERS TO SIMULATION EDUCATION

As with any new learning tool there are often barriers to change. The integration of simulation into the curricula of nursing and other health care fields is no exception. The identification of such barriers can help lead to change. Cost is often a significant barrier to simulation education. Although models for implementation exist, limited information is available about adopting high-technology simulation when cost and resources are significant barriers.[20] In 2010 Adamson[21] surveyed associate degree nursing programs to identify barriers to simulation use. Adamson discovered faculty noted that "helpful and thorough training in the use of simulation" was an obstacle when attempting to fully use simulation pedagogy. Masunaga and Hitchcock[22] pointed out that "faculty failed to exhibit such congruence for the following descriptions of an ideal clinical teachers: stimulating, well-read, and innovative." Taplay and colleagues[23] in their article about strategies used by nursing leaders to shape the adoption and incorporation of simulation into nursing curricula comment that nursing leaders and administrators must overcome the barriers of human and financial resources by working together to negotiate, navigate, and network to have a true impact on the integration of simulation into the curricula. Barjis[24] comments that "user resistance is a major barrier to a successful simulation implementation in healthcare. [This] barrier exists in concert with the fact that simulation, especially detailed simulation, requires tremendous effort and time."

One noted obstruction to simulation faculty development has been the lack of standards or competencies.[25] In 2011 the International Nursing Association for Clinical Simulation and Learning (INACSL) adopted a set of simulation standards that are beginning to be incorporated within nursing simulation programs across the country. The introduction of these much needed standards has helped provide some guidance and structure to faculty education. To become proficient, faculty must "continually review their understanding of good teaching and integrate such understanding into their core existence."[22] Simulation nurse educators are no exception and should demand their programs follow best educational evidence.

CURRENT TRENDS: PROFESSIONAL ORGANIZATIONS

The emergence of professional organizations that provide education for simulation educators has begun to meet a great need in terms of educational opportunities for faculty. The INACSL has grown from a grass roots organization originally begun to support nursing educators in laboratory settings in the 1990s to the robust group of simulation experts that currently are a part of this vital group. In 2011 INACSL released the first standards of best practice that provided a framework for simulation educators when implementing simulation pedagogy. Since 2011 INACSL has updated the standards of practice and is a leader providing a much needed foundation for educating faculty in the use of simulation. In addition to INACSL, the Society for Simulation in Healthcare (SSIH) has become a leader in the interprofessional support for simulation faculty and staff. The SSIH has developed an accreditation process for faculty and organizations to recognize experts in simulation education. Although these organizations are vital to the support of simulation in health care education, not all faculty and staff have the fiscal ability to join these groups or attend annual conferences.

On a more local level there has been an emergence of statewide alliances that support local education and often provide a more affordable solution for educators and institutions. In California, the California Simulation Alliance (CSA) (http://www.californiasimulationalliance.org/) provides registered nurses and other health care professionals with a virtual collaborative that "enhances and fosters" simulation development. The director of the CAS supports the "development of a solid, comprehensive curriculum [that] allows the program to be replicated in other areas of the state. The common language, standards, and consistency of the curriculum [allow the CSA] to develop a critical mass of simulation users that share the same goals and philosophy regarding simulation education."[19] Another strong alliance funded through the Florida Center for Nursing and Blue Care is the Florida Simulation Alliance (FSA) (http://www.floridahealthsimalliance.org/Home.aspx), which aims to help with the advancement, coordination, and expansion of simulation in the academic and health care settings. The FSA has identified opportunities for instructor development through workshops and conference offerings. "Development of a workshop series for instructors at both basic and advanced levels, based on common simulation principles, is an opportunity to address this need."[26] Funding for such alliances has been the key to their long-term success and sustainability and often makes them more affordable for local educators. Other states, such as Oregon (http://www.oregonsimulation.com/), Virginia (http://www.virginiasimulationallianceinc.org/), and Tennessee (http://tnsim.org/), have alliances that offer a reasonable option for educational offerings. These alliances also promote sharing of information among educators and the beginning of interprofessional activities.

CURRENT TRENDS: OTHER

One of the most often cited barriers to simulation is the education and support for simulation faculty and staff. In addition to the aforementioned organizations there have emerged some innovative groups that provide free and/or reasonably priced simulation materials. The University of Washington Center for Health Sciences Inter-professional Education, Research and Practice has developed World Wide Web resources that are open to the public through a Health Resources and Health Admin-istration grant. The resources are peer reviewed and provide detailed information on simulation education (http://collaborate.uw.edu/faculty-development/teaching-with-simulation/teaching-with-simulation.html-0). Another valuable resource comes from a joint venture from the National League for Nursing and vendor support from Laerdal Medical, the Simulation Innovation Resource Center (SIRC) found online at http://sirc.nln.org/. This SIRC site is noted to be an innovative online resource that provides webinars, online courses, and forums to discuss simulation pedagogy and faculty development. There are many other valuable online resources available to those seeking to learn more about simulation.

FACULTY TRAINING: WHAT, WHERE, HOW, AND WHEN?

The previously discussed resources are crucial to the further implementation of simu-lation education. However, examining more closely what nursing educators are doing to provide faculty development also provides great insight into how simulation faculty can be educated. Considering the facilitator (faculty) in simulation education and the training of such is imperative. The facilitator monitors and assists students as they strive to comprehend and reach the simulation and curricular outcomes. "In addition, the facilitator engages the participants to search for evidence-based practice solu-tions in order to develop the participant's skill development and clinical judgment."[27] In the 2013 revision of the INACSL standards, there is a clear statement regarding training the facilitator: "the facilitator has specific simulation education provided by formal coursework, continuing education offerings, and targeted work with an experi-enced mentor."[28] As with all learning, the implementation of what one has learned can be fostered by working alongside or having input from an expert or mentor.

Several barriers to simulation education were identified earlier. In a 2009 study Jansen and coworkers[29] noted that barriers to simulation prevented faculty from using simulation effectively and thus negatively impacted student learning. The team subse-quently identified areas that impacted faculty acceptance of simulation: time, training, attitude, lack of space and equipment, scheduling of the laboratory, funding, staffing, and engaging students.[29] Training in each of these areas can help facilitate the suc-cessful implementation of simulation across the spectrum. Each of these areas iden-tified can be addressed through the training of faculty and the intentional planning of simulation integration.

Included within the INACSL 2013 revision of the standards are the following topics, and each of these standards must be included in faculty development plans[30]:

Standard I: Terminology – provide consistency
Standard II: Professional integrity of participants
Standard III: Participant objectives – clear and measurable
Standard IV: Facilitation – multiple methods
Standard V: Facilitator – proficiency
Standard VI: Debriefing process – improve practice through reflection
Standard VII: Participant assessment and evaluation

EDUCATION

Nurse faculty often experience "curricular creep," which is described as the addition of more and more material into a nursing curriculum. The addition of simulation technology to the tools used to teach is often overwhelming (time to learn to use new technology proficiently) and faculty may feel like this is an additional task that needs to be completed. Simulation cannot simply be added into the curricula. Faculty must together develop a plan of implementation. The National Council of State Boards of Nursing study released in 2014[31] supports the use of simulation to replace some clinical experiences (hours); using simulation to replace a portion of the required hours varies from state to state. However, the use of simulation should not be added into the already crowded requirements without a significant review of the curriculum by all involved. Taplay and coworkers[23] describe this process as "finding a fit"; where can simulation be used effectively, aligning with "the courses and curricula...in addition, reflection on the capability of the equipment to meet the course and curricular learning objectives" is essential. Jansen and coworkers[29] support faculty training and meeting the time obstacle through creative use of graduate students, sharing scenarios with colleagues, and professional networking. An important common theme seen in the literature is the identification of a "champion" within the nursing faculty. This person may or may not be officially identified as the simulation champion but can be "pivotal to the actualization of the vision of integrating simulation throughout the curriculum."[32]

Faculty training can be overwhelming. As early as 2008 Jeffries[33] identified the need for educator preparation in simulation. Jeffries[33] described four essential elements (STEP) to simulation faculty training: Standardization of materials, Train the trainer, Encourage simulation design and implementation team, and Plan to coordinate simulation development and implementation.[33]

Since her publication there have been multiple attempts to provide regional simulation education along with simulation publications related to summer institutes, faculty workshops, and annual requirements.[1,23,34] There is not one best method identified to provide simulation education for faculty and staff. However, the INACSL standards provide an essential framework to model educational offerings.[30] Intentional education based on INACSL standards is an ideal place to begin. An essential first step is to ensure faculty have a basic understanding of how equipment and technology works.[29] This basic understanding can be met through vendor training; however, it is important that further education related to pedagogy and theory be subsequent next steps. INACSL standards include common terminology simulation educators must be familiar with to be proficient to understand current evidence surrounding simulation pedagogy and to provide consistency within faculty facilitators. All of the standards are important to the effective use of simulation and scant evidence has been published related to the most important topics in which faculty need to be educated. Taibi and Kardong-Edgren[1] noted in their online survey that most faculty seek training related specifically to debriefing and simulation development.

SUMMARY

Although there still remains much discussion on how to train faculty in simulation, the development of standards for faculty training and certifications for simulation educators is a positive move toward consistency. Much work remains to get nurse educators to a level of proficiency with simulation education. We must applaud those nurse educators who have been innovators in the education and training of others and pay close attention to best evidence as the research continues to emerge.

REFERENCES

1. Taibi DM, Kardong-Edgren S. Health care educator training in simulation: a survey and web site development. Clinical Simulation in Nursing 2014;10(1): e47–52.
2. Bargagliotti L. President's message. The DNP: historical parallels and persistent questions. Nursing Education Perspectives [serial online] 2006;27(4):174. Available from: CINAHL Plus with Full Text, Ipswich, MA. Accessed April 12, 2015.
3. Poindexter K. Perceived essential novice nurse educator role competencies and qualifications to teach in a pre-licensure registered nurse education program [doctoral dissertation]. Kalamazoo (MI): Western Michigan University; 2008.
4. American Association of Colleges of Nursing. AACN applauds the new Carnegie Foundation report calling for a more highly educated nursing workforce. 2010. Available at: http://www.aacn.nche.edu/news/articles/2010/carnegie.
5. Benner P, Leonard V, Day L. Book highlights from educating nurses: a call for radical transformation. carnegie; 2010. Available at: http://archive.carnegiefoundation.org/elibrary/educating-nurses-highlights.
6. Institute of Medicine. To err is human: building a safer health system. IOM; 1999.
7. James JT. A new, evidence-based estimate of patient harms associated with hospital care. J Patient Saf 2013;9(3):122–8.
8. Department of Health Policy and Management U.S. Senate Committee on Health Education, Labor and Pensions Subcommittee on Primary Health and Aging. Testimony of Ashish K. Jha, MD, MPH, Professor of Health Policy and Management, Harvard School of Public Health. 2014. Available at: http://www.help.senate.gov/imo/media/doc/Jha.pdf.
9. Seropian MA, Brown K, Gavilanes JS, et al. Simulation: not just a manikin. J Nurs Educ 2004;43(4):164–9.
10. Alexander M. Effectiveness of traditional clinical and simulation experiences. J Nurs Regul 2014;5(3):3.
11. Seybert AL. Patient simulation in pharmacy education. Am J Pharm Educ 2011; 75(9):187.
12. Peters M. Does constructivist epistemology have a place in nurse education? J Nurs Educ 2000;39(4):166–72.
13. American Association of Colleges and Universities. Taking responsibility for the quality of the baccalaureate degree. 2004.
14. American Association of Colleges of Nursing. The essentials of baccalaureate education for professional nursing practice. 2008.
15. Meyer C, Jones TB. Promoting active learning: strategies for the college classroom. Jossey Bass, Inc; 1993.
16. Jeffries PR. Technology trends in nursing education: next steps. J Nurs Educ 2006;44(1):3–4.
17. Burgess CC. Developing a collaborative regional nursing simulation hospital. Teach Learn Nurs 2007;2(2):53–7.
18. Decker SI. Simulation as an educational strategy in the development of critical and reflective thinking: a qualitative exploration. Ann Arbor (MI): Texas Woman's University; 2007.
19. Waxman KT, Telles CL. The use of Benner's framework in high-fidelity simulation faculty development: the bay area simulation collaborative model. Clinical Simulation in Nursing 2009;5(6):e231–5.
20. Curtin MM, Dupuis MD. Development of human patient simulation programs: achieving big results with a small budget. J Nurs Educ 2008;47(11):522–3.

21. Adamson K. Integrating human patient simulation into associate degree nursing curricula. Clinical Simulation in Nursing 2010;6(3):e75–81.
22. Masunaga H, Hitchcock MA. Aligning teaching practices with an understanding of quality teaching: a faculty development agenda. Med Teach 2011;33(2): 124–30.
23. Taplay K, Jack SM, Baxter P, et al. Negotiating, navigating, and networking: three strategies used by nursing leaders to shape the adoption and incorporation of simulation into nursing curricula—a grounded theory study. ISRN Nurs 2014;2014:7.
24. Barjis J. Healthcare simulation and its potential areas and future trends. SCS M&S Magazine 2011;2011(1):6.
25. Ng G. Championing faculty development. The nurse education imperative. Nurs Econ 2013;31(1):42.
26. Sole ML, Guimond ME, Amidei C. An analysis of simulation resources, needs, and plans in Florida. Clinical Simulation in Nursing 2013;9(7):e265–71.
27. Directors. Standard V: simulation facilitator. Clinical simulation in nursing 2013; 7(4):S14–5.
28. Boese T, Cato M, Gonzalez L, et al. Standards of best practice: simulation standard V: facilitator. Clinical Simulation in Nursing 2013;9(6):S22–5.
29. Jansen DA, Johnson N, Larson G, et al. Nursing faculty perceptions of obstacles to utilizing manikin-based simulations and proposed solutions. Clinical Simulation in Nursing 2009;5(1):e9–16.
30. Directors. Standards of best practice: simulation. Clinical Simulation in Nursing 2013;9(6 Supplement):ii–iii.
31. Jennifer KH, Smiley RA, Alexander M, et al. The NCSBN national simulation study: a longitudinal, randomized, controlled study replacing clinical hours with simulation in prelicensure nursing education. J Nurs Regul 2014;5(2):S2–64.
32. Conrad MA, Guhde J, Brown D, et al. Transformational leadership: instituting a nursing simulation program. Clinical Simulation in Nursing 2011;7(5):e189–95.
33. Jeffries PR. Getting in S.T.E.P. with simulations: simulations take educator preparation. Nurs Educ Perspect 2008;29(2):70–3.
34. Jones AL, Fahrenwald N, Ficek A. Testing Ajzen's theory of planned behavior for faculty simulation development. Clinical Simulation in Nursing 2013;9(6):e213–8.

Thinking of Serving Nursing Abroad

How Technology Assists Nurses on Mission Trips

Rachel M. Brown, CRNA, DNP

KEYWORDS

- Short-term mission • International • Nurse • Nurse anesthesia • Faith-based
- Technology

KEY POINTS

- Know yourself and be open to change. Individuals who desire to participate in short-term missions need to be sure their personal world-view aligns with the sponsoring organization.
- Collaborate with those who have gone before you. There is no need to reinvent the wheel. The experience of others is of great benefit.
- Prepare, prepare, prepare. Communicate with your group members in advance, pack efficiently, and prepare to enjoy a life-changing experience.

INTRODUCTION

Advances in technology have assisted in the proliferation of short-term, faith-based international medical mission trips in the twenty-first century. Mission trips vary and include combinations of providing health care, building homes, churches and schools, and sharing the Gospel.[1] Other services may also include training local health care professionals, education[2,3] and "ongoing support for leadership development".[3] Technological advances have improved the logistics associated with the planning, preparation, and implementation of international short-term, faith-based missions. Health care and international Christian missionary journeys are now far removed from days of ocean-liner travel across the seas, days and weeks of travel by horseback, and weeks or months without communication to the outside world. However, after arrival to a remote area of a third-world country, one may be asked to perform health care without the resources to which the provider may be accustomed.

Disclosure statement: The author has nothing to disclose.
Middle Tennessee School of Anesthesia, 315 Hospital Drive, Madison, TN 37116, USA
E-mail address: Rachel.brown@mtsa.edu

Nurs Clin N Am 50 (2015) 399–410
http://dx.doi.org/10.1016/j.cnur.2015.02.005
0029-6465/15/$ – see front matter © 2015 Elsevier Inc. All rights reserved.

nursing.theclinics.com

DISCUSSION: MY STORY

I began my nursing career in 1986 and it has included intensive care nursing (ICU) medical-surgical nursing, and home health nursing. Following graduation from a school of nurse anesthesia in 1997, my career as a Certified Registered Nurse Anesthetist (CRNA) began. Twelve years later I returned to school and completed my Doctor of Nursing Practice (DNP) degree. I then transitioned into the academic world of nurse anesthesia education, where I am now an Assistant Program Administrator. Following this career transition I became intensely drawn to the vast world of international short-term, faith-based missions.

The mission statement and core values of the school of anesthesia where I am employed closely align with my own personal Christian values and mission focus. The following is a summation of the mission statement:

We assist nurse anesthesia students in the pursuit of truth and learning to become the best they can be, and to give back and develop a life-long commitment to serving others.

The mission statement embraces a life of service that also aligns with my personal desire to exercise my Christian faith and serve others. There is a great demand for volunteer Registered Nurses[4,5] and Certified Registered Nurse Anesthetists (CRNAs) to be involved in international short-term, faith-based mission trips. I have now developed a formal program for my school to support the Mission Statement of a life-long commitment to serve others.

HOW DOES ONE BEGIN A FORMAL MISSION PROGRAM?

There are multiple steps in beginning a formal mission program (**Box 1**). In the remainder of the article I will describe in detail the steps to begin a formal mission program.

Step One: Collaboration with Others Who Have Traveled and Experienced International Short-Term, Faith-Based Medical Missions

Collaboration is defined as working with another person or group in order to achieve or do something.[5,6] To collaborate with an experienced short-term

---

Box 1
Beginning a formal mission program: personal experience

1. Collaboration with others who have traveled and experienced international short-term, faith-based medical mission.

2. Obtain permission to travel with an existing experienced team.

3. Establish email, phone, and/or video-conferencing communication to be up to date on trip information/travel changes

4. Begin personal financial planning/fundraising for trip

5. Obtain necessary medical documentation/immunizations

6. Obtain necessary passport documents

7. Be flexible. Circumstances can change unexpectedly.

After you are an experienced short-term mission traveler:

8. Present proposal for short-term mission program to appropriate Dept. at your institution

mission participant, I called a colleague who is a Program Director at a faith-based school of nurse anesthesia. She is experienced in mission trips and has led many groups on international short-term mission trips. I was invited to travel with her group of student registered nurse anesthetists (SRNAs) on their next trip. We had multiple conversations via phone, email, and text. I also perused the internet and found numerous website listings of both faith-based and nonreligious humanitarian mission groups (**Box 2**). Other tips for promoting good collaboration include:

- Find an organization/school whose mission most closely aligns with your own beliefs and goals.[7–11]
- Research the organization with whom you are collaborating.[7,8,12]
- Contact friends or family who have traveled on similar mission trips.[1]

Link to website for multiple listings: www.missionfinder.org.

Box 2
Websites for faith-based, and non faith-based based short-term medical mission organizations

Faith Medical Missions	www.faithmed.org
Catholic Medical Mission Board	www.cmmb.org
Christian Aid	www.christianaid.org.uk
For Haiti	www.forhaitiwithlove.org
Mercy Ships	www.mercyships.org
The Salvation Army World Service	www.sawso.org
SCORE International	www.scoreintl.org
LiveBeyond	www.livebeyond.org
Impact Ministries	www.impactministriesusa.org
Missionary Ventures International	www.mvi.org
Volunteers In Medical Missions	www.vimm.org
Partners in Progress	www.partnersinprogress.org
Volunteers in Service Abroad (VISA)	www.visaministries.org
Samaritans Purse	www.samaritanspurse.org
Christian Medical and Dental Association	www.cmda.org
Project Hope	www.projecthope.org
Mercy and Truth Medical Missions	www.mercyandtruth.com
Christian Health Service Corps	www.medicalmissions.com
Christian Medical Mission, Inc	www.christianmedical.org
Baptist Medical and Dental Missions International	www.bmdi.org
Operation Smile (non-faith based)	www.operationsmile.org
Doctors Without Borders (non-faith based)	www.doctorswithoutborders.org

This list is by no means all inclusive. It is intended only as a guide.

Step Two: Obtain Permission/Authorization to Travel with an Existing Experienced Team

Although my colleague was agreeable that I join their next mission trip to the Dominican Republic, I first had to obtain permission from her Dean of the School of Nursing, since I was not one of their students or faculty. Permission was granted, and preparation began to join this nurse anesthesia team which included CRNAs and Student Registered Nurse Anesthetists (SRNAs).

For my second mission trip, I was more informed due to my prior experience. I chose to partner with an established Christian faith-based group to visit in Haiti. Technology was supportive in an easy on-line registration. Due to a shortage of nursing volunteers for a mission, I was asked to participate in March instead of May. Because of my first trip, my passport and vaccinations were current, and I was able to travel 2 months earlier than originally planned.

In the same calendar year, I was asked to join a non-government organization (NGO) and travel to Cambodia. Again, on-line registration, communication, and exchange of information were relatively easy due to all our state-side technology. This particular NGO needed a CRNA to provide anesthesia services, and to be an ambassador of sorts to the local military anesthesia providers. United States (U.S.) military personnel were also volunteers on this mission. Collaboration and sharing good-will between members of the Cambodian military and volunteers from the U.S. were the focus of the mission.

Suggestions for obtaining permission to join with a mission group include:

- Make sure you have documented permission from key authoritative personnel associated with the mission trip.
- Verify with family members that they support your travel. Do not surprise them.
- Verify time away from work with your employer and get permission in writing, to avoid last minute miscommunication.
- Take notes about the logistics and planning process for the group.
- Learn from others experiences what has worked well and what has not worked well.
- Remember that you are a guest with the group and in the country you are visiting. Be courteous and professional.

Step Three: Establish Communication with Mission Group Leadership

Communication with the leaders of the mission group was an important part of being accepted into an existing mission program. I requested my name to be added to the email list of students and faculty from the school of anesthesia that would be traveling together. Email communication allowed me to begin to learn the names of everyone in the group, and for them to learn a little information about me. Suggestions for items to pack were discussed within each group with whom I traveled (**Box 3**). The packing lists were similar, however each country visited specified certain items unique to that location (**Table 1**). For example, in both the Dominican and Haiti locations I had to bring my own bath linens. In Cambodia those amenities were provided. I stayed in a nice, urban hotel. Besides not to over-pack, some other pearls I learned from my experiences include:

- Carefully read all communications from the group leader. They have experience and you do not.
- Write down any questions you may have before sending multiple emails, or making multiple phone calls.
- Meet all required deadlines. Do not be late with registration, turning in documents, or making payments. This is courteous and professional behavior, and late can equate to not being accepted to travel.
- Keep all communication positive, professional, and timely.

Box 3
Sample packing list (compiled from several lists. Items will vary depending on country/area visited)

Passport and VISA (make copies)

Passport carrier (either around your neck or waist)

Money belt

Backpack for day travel

Comfortable close-toed shoes

Underwear/socks for each day

Scrubs for each day

Multiple T-shirts

Sleeping clothes (to be in a room with others)

Earplugs (if snoring bothers you)

Flashlight and extra batteries

Camera, charger and extra batteries

Phone and charger

Toiletries

Medications (personal Rx)

Prevention meds (diarrhea, motion sickness, headache, etc)

Adhesive bandage strips

Bath linens

Deet (90% plus if in malaria prone region)

Anti-malaria Rx

Hand sanitizer and body wipes

Sunscreen

Sunglasses

Extra pair of prescription eye glasses

Hat

Watch

Snacks

Powder flavor packets for water

Bible and journal

Emergency toilet paper

Bed linens/small pillow

Step Four: Financial Planning/Fundraising

Priest and Priest found that the average cost of an international short-term mission trip was between $1001 to $1450.[13] In 2013, the cost of my first mission trip to the Dominican Republic was $1800. This included round-trip airfare, in-country transportation, lodging, meals, travel health insurance, and fees paid to translators. There were additional costs: updating passport, vaccinations, international cell phone service, snacks,

Table 1	
Links to websites for immunization information	
Centers for Disease Control and Prevention	www.cdc.gov
Passport Health USA	www.PassportHealthUSA.com
American Society of Travel Medicine and Hygiene	www.astmh.org
International Society of Travel Medicine	www.istm.org
Costco	www.costco.com
CVS Pharmacies	www.cvs.com
Kroger Pharmacies	www.kroger.com
Walgreens Pharmacies	www.walgreens.com
Wal-Mart Pharmacies	www.walmart.com
Target Pharmacies	www.target.com

and souvenirs. Individuals need to be aware of the full cost of a short-term mission trip prior to committing to participating.[14,15] The cost of my mission trip to Haiti, as well as Cambodia, was approximately $2000. Fundraising for your trip should begin earlier rather than later. The first group with which I collaborated provided a standardized letter for fundraising (Appendix).

Step Five: Obtain Necessary Medical Documentation and Immunizations

Travel to third world countries and other under-developed locations raises health concerns for those entering these medically underserved regions. For personal safety, and the safety of the mission team, there must be a review of each participant's current immunization status and the need for additional immunizations. Furthermore, a complete health screening should be completed to make sure the participant is healthy enough for travel and strenuous activity.[14–17] Proper immunization can help reduce the risk of preventable infectious disease to the health care providers as well as preventing bringing the disease into the U.S.[18] The Centers for Disease Control and Prevention (CDC) website provides valuable information related to what vaccines may be needed, dependent upon the region being visited.[16] Additional resources include travel medicine clinics. Passport Health USA is a nationwide travel medicine clinic that offers immunizations and education related to international travel.[19] The CDC currently recommends all routine immunizations be up to date, with the additional vaccines for Hepatitis A, Hepatitis B, and tetanus. Travel to some areas may require vaccination against Typhoid and Yellow Fever.[16] The American Society of Tropical Medicine and Hygiene provides an on-line medicine consultant directory. This directory is a "list of physicians who offer clinical consultive service in tropical medicine, medical parasitology and travelers' health".[20] Refer to **Table 1** for links to websites for immunization information. Using the technology of the internet, mission teams can search for local providers in their community. The web-based search may also provide information for cost comparison of immunizations.

Step Six: Obtain Necessary Passport and Visa Documents

Although this step seems less complicated than those above, obtaining or updating a passport does not happen overnight. In fact, the process can take months to complete. Each of the mission groups with which I have traveled required passport documents to have an expiration date at least 6 months past return to the United States. My mission trip to Cambodia required a travel/work VISA. To obtain the VISA, my passport had to be current and mailed to the appropriate government agency well in advance of my trip. The NGO with which I was working made all of the arrangements, but there was still a concern about time for return of the documents for travel.

It is also important to make extra copies of your VISA and Passport. Leave copies with family members at home, and keep copies, along with the originals, tucked away in a safe place on your person while you travel.[14,21,22] If the originals are lost during your travel, you can have your family members fax, email, or text message photos of your documents for the local embassy to process.

Link to United States passport information
U.S. Department of State: Bureau of Consular Affairs http://travel.state.gov/content/travel/english.html.

Step Seven: Be Flexible. Circumstances Can Change Unexpectedly

Every mission trip I participated in had some unexpected circumstance occur. The small hospital in the Dominican Republic at which we were to provide anesthesia had no EKG stickers, and only one tank of medical oxygen was available for two operating suites. We also had to resort to cleaning the only available nasal cannula with 70% alcohol between patient use. The team of CRNAs and SRNAs were still able to provide anesthesia services, but the limited amount of oxygen also restricted the use of general anesthesia. Regional anesthesia became the method most utilized that week. Supplies and equipment can be limited to non-existant. Review with team leaders the supplies and equipment required to perform safe and accurate care, just as you would in the U.S. Companies exist that can donate some of the necessary supplies prior to your departure: for example Project Cure www.project.cure.org.

Services provided the week in Haiti included treatment for scabies, urinary tract infections, ear infections, and upper respiratory infections (**Figs.1–4**).

Our team also monitored patients for malnutrition, a prevalent problem in remote regions of Haiti. Bags of beans and rice were given to those patients whose body-mass-index (BMI) was below 17. Minor cuts and abrasions were cleaned and bandaged. One child who had suffered a severe burn on her arm was brought to the clinic by her mother. She returned each day for debridement of the wound and clean bandages (**Fig. 5**).

Step Eight: Present Proposal at Your Institution for Implementation of Short-term Mission Program

Presenting my proposal for the implementation of an international short-term faith-based mission program proved to be relatively simple. A key element was to provide factual information to the academic committee regarding:

- Costs
- Time commitment
- The logistics of preparing students for a mission trip

During my three medical mission trips in 2014, I had gathered a wealth of information about planning, preparation, and implementation of such a program. In addition to the logistics portion of the presentation, my overwhelming enthusiasm and personal commitment was evident as well. The academic committee at my institution gave full consent for the implementation of an international short-term, faith-based

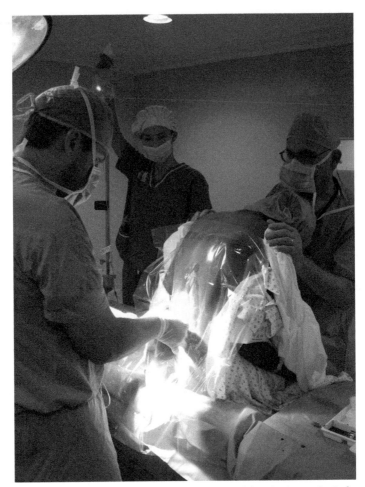

Fig. 1. Under the supervision of CRNA faculty, SRNAs provide spinal anesthetic for a patient in the Dominican Republic, 2014.

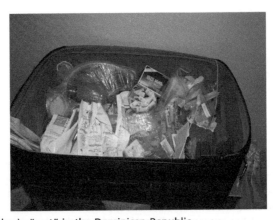

Fig. 2. Our anesthesia "cart" in the Dominican Republic.

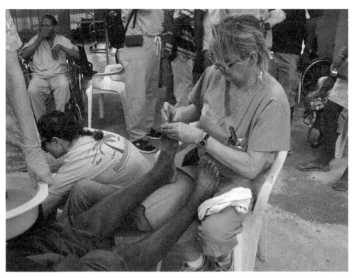

Fig. 3. The author Rachel Brown, CRNA, provided hand and foot care to nursing home residents in the Dominican Republic. Mission participants must be flexible to provide for the needs of the local citizens.

mission program. Our first trip with a group of our nurse anesthesia students will occur in 2015.

1. Show your enthusiasm for the program
2. Provide a well organized packet with pictures for committee members to reference.
3. Be factual in the presentation.

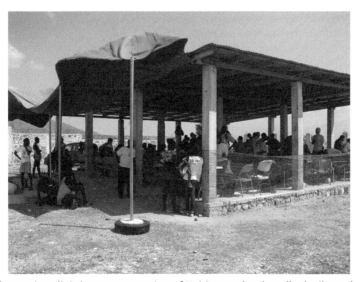

Fig. 4. The nursing clinic in a remote region of Haiti: some locals walked miles to be seen at the clinic.

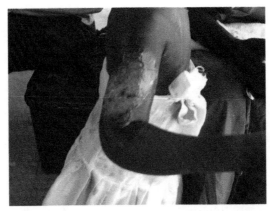

Fig. 5. Young child in Haiti who was treated for a severe burn on her arm.

SUMMARY: TECHNOLOGICAL DIFFERENCES FOR THE AMERICAN CRNA PARTICIPATING IN INTERNATIONAL SHORT-TERM FAITH-BASED MEDICAL MISSIONS; A PERSONAL PERSPECTIVE

- Language barriers exist. Reliance on local translators was key to successful patient/provider interaction. Be prepared to pay translators.
- Be creative with technology. Use cell phones or computer tablets to access photos/diagrams to aid with the explanation of procedures to patients.
- Electronic translation devices may not always have the correct pronunciation, and may not be 100% reliable.
- Cell phones and computer tablets do not always work in third-world or developing countries, due to limited cell phone towers and satellite coverage.
- Regions that lack health care personnel will most likely be lacking in supplies as well. More than 90% of the anesthesia supplies we used were brought to the site from donations by American hospitals.
- Charting and record keeping will be old-school paper and pen. An organized medical chart may be non-existent.
- Be flexible. Although I am a CRNA, the majority of my time spent on medical mission trips has been spent providing basic first-aid, general nursing care, and prayer with those who had spiritual needs.
- Be quiet and patient. Observe and learn from cultures much different from your own. This does not require batteries or any special technological device.

REFERENCES

1. Venable H. Anesthesia on a medical mission to Guatemala. Plast Surg Nurs 2005; 25(3):129–32. Available at: http://journals.lww.com/psnjournalonline/Citation/2005/07000/Anesthesia_on_a_Medical_Mission_to_Guatemala.7.aspx. Accessed October 2, 2014.
2. Riviello R, Ozgediz D, Hsia RY, et al. Role of collaborative academic partnerships in surgical training, education, and provision. World J Surg 2010;34:459–65.
3. Gill Z, Carlough M. Do mission hospitals have a role in achieving Millennium Development Goal 5? Int J Gynaecol Obstet 2008;102(2):198–202. Available at: http://www.ijgo.org/article/S0020-7292(08)00156-2/pdf. Accessed October 1, 2014.

4. Senior K. Wanted: 2.4 million nurses, and that's just in India. Bull World Health Organ 2010;88(5):327–8. Available at: http://www.who.int/bulletin/volumes/88/5/10-020510/en/#. Accessed December 12, 2014.

5. Beal JA. Academic service partnerships in nursing: an integrative review. Nurs Res Pract 2012;2012:501564.

6. Merriam-Webster Dictionary. Merriam-Webster Dictionary Web site. Available at: http://www.merriam-webster.com/dictionary/collaboration. Accessed October 5, 2014.

7. Chahine E, Nornoo A. Pharmacist involvement in medical missions: Planning, execution, and assessment. Am J Health Syst Pharm 2012;69(8):636, 638, 640, 642–3.

8. Kolkin JA. physician's perspective on volunteering overseas...It's not all about sharing the latest technology. J Hand Ther 2014;27:152–7. Available at: http://dx.doi.org/10.1016/j.jht.2013.09.002. Accessed October 2, 2014.

9. Chapin E, Doocy S. International short-term medical service trips: guidelines from the literature and perspectives from the field. World Health Popul 2010;12(2): 43–53.

10. Suchdev P, Ahrens K, Click E, et al. A model for sustainable short-term international medical trips. Ambul Pediatr 2007;7(4):317–20.

11. Brown DA, Ferrill MJ. Planning a pharmacy-led medical mission trip, part 1: focus on medication acquisition. Ann Pharmacother 2014;46:751–9.

12. Solheim J, Edwards P. Planning a successful mission trip: the ins and outs. J Emerg Nurs 2007;33(4):382–7.

13. Priest RJ, Priest JP. They see everything, and understand nothing: short-term mission and service learning. Missiology 2008;36(1):53–73. Available at: http://mis.sagepub.com/content/36/1/53. Accessed October 1, 2014.

14. Chapman C. So you want to go on a medical mission? J Nurs Pract 2007;3(10): 707–12.

15. Birman MV, Kolkin J. How to volunteer overseas. J Hand Surg 2013;38(A):802–3. Available at: http://dx.doi.org/10.1016/j.jhsa.2012.12.040. Accessed October 1, 2014.

16. Centers for Disease Control and Prevention: travelers health. Centers for Disease Control Web site. Available at: http://wwwnc.cdc.gov/Travel. Accessed October 2, 2014.

17. Stoney R, Jentes ES, Sotir MJ, et al. Global TravEpiNet. Pre-travel preparation of US travelers going abroad to provide humanitarian service, Global TravEpiNet 2001-2011. Am J Trop Med Hyg 2014;90(3):553–9.

18. Leggat PA. Routine vaccinations and travel. In: Wilder-Smith A, Schwartz E, Shaw M, editors. Travel medicine tales behind the science. Amsterdam: Elsevier; 2007. p. 39–46.

19. Passport Health. Passport Health USA Web site. Available at: http://www.passporthealthusa.com/locations/tn/brentwood/395/. Accessed October 5, 2014.

20. The American Society of Tropical Medicine and Hygiene. The American Society of Tropical Medicine and Hygiene Web site. Available at: http://www.astmh.org//AM/Template.cfm?Section=Home1. Accessed October 5, 2014.

21. United States Department of State: Bureau of Consular Affairs. US Department of State Web site. Available at: http://travel.state.gov/content/travel/english.html. Accessed October 5, 2014.

22. Project Cure Web site. Available at: www.projectcure.org. Accessed January 20, 2015.

APPENDIX: SAMPLE FUNDRAISING LETTER

{Date}
{Name}
{Address}
{City, State}
Dear _____,

I hope this letter finds you well. As you know, I am currently a graduate nursing student in the Nurse Anesthesia track at XXXXX. One goal of the program is to provide an opportunity for each student to use their God given knowledge and skills on a short-term mission trip.

From January 25 through February 2, 2014, faculty from the School of Nursing –Nurse Anesthesia track will be taking me with them on a mission trip to the Dominican Republic. The ultimate purpose of this mission trip will be to share the gospel and allow God to speak to my heart while allowing me to serve on a team providing medical services in a hospital providing anesthesia services for approximately 50 surgical patients, followed by venturing into remote areas of the Dominican Republic to provide healthcare services in community-based clinics.

In being able to serve on this team, I am asking for your financial support. While the total cost of the trip will be approximately $ 1800, I am asking if you can provide support for any portion of the total cost. Your financial support for this trip will not only allow me to serve God's children in the Dominican Republic, but allow God to speak to me during a time of stillness and worship.

Checks made out to XXXXXX will be considered tax-deductible gifts and donors will receive a receipt from XXXXXX. Donations should go to: *INSERT NAME AND ADDRESS OF INDIVIDUAL.*

Her e-mail address is XXXXXX phone number is XXXXXXXX. Please write my name somewhere on the check so she will know how to credit your contribution. Donations are due by November 15, 2013.

As a point of clarity, your contribution is being given to the School of Nursing at XXXXXXXX. If for some reason I am not able to go on the trip, your contribution will remain in the nursing fund to be used for other mission opportunities under the School of Nursing at the discretion of the Office of International Missions.

Thank you for your prayerful consideration and I look forward to telling you how God impacted my life when I return from the mission trip. If you have further questions and desire to speak with the mission trip team leader, please contact XXXXXXXXX, Chair of the Nurse Anesthesia Track at XXXXXXXX or XXXXXXXX, Asst. Chair of the Nurse Anesthesia Track at XXXXXXXX.

God bless,

{signature}

{name}

Courtesy of Union University, Jackson, Tennessee; with permission.

Perioperative Nurses' Knowledge of Indicators for Pressure Ulcer Development in the Surgical Patient Population

CrossMark

Susan Krauser Lupear, DNP, CRNA, APRN[a],*,
Maria Overstreet, PhD, RN[b,c], Stephen D. Krau, PhD, RN, CNE[c]

KEYWORDS

- Technology in surgery • Pressure ulcers • Ulcer measurement scale • Nursing
- Perioperative nursing

KEY POINTS

- More than 2 million people in the United States experience the effects of pressure ulcers (PUs) each year. It is estimated that less than 5% of patients admitted to the hospital develop a PU; however, this percentage increases to more than 45% once patients are admitted to the perioperative area. The financial expenditure for health care for patients who have developed a PU ranges from $750 million to greater than $1 billion.
- Although assessment tools have proved to be beneficial in certain patient populations, there is a question about the accuracy and sensitivity of the assessment tools for the risk of PU development in the surgical patient population. The overall score a patient receives on the assessment tool predicts the extent to which the patient is at risk for PU development.
- Perioperative nurses are often the initial health care providers for the surgical patient population because they prepare patients for surgical procedures. In that most PUs are preventable, perioperative nurses play a pivotal role in the prevention of PU development.
- Specific surgical procedures and patient factors were identified as indicators for PU development in surgical patients and include intraoperative patient temperature, length of surgical procedure, patient position required for surgery, hemoglobin and hematocrit levels, hemodynamic stability, preoperative albumin level, and comorbidities (eg, diabetes mellitus and peripheral vascular disease). In addition, the use of vasoactive medications to support blood pressure can increase the incidence of PU development in surgical patients by 33%. Incorporating patient-specific and surgical procedure–specific indicators that place surgical patients at risk for developing PUs is essential to ensure the prevention of PU development.

Disclosure: None.
[a] Vanderbilt University Medical Center, Nashville, TN, USA; [b] Center for Clinical Simulation, Middle Tennessee School of Anesthesia, Madison, TN, USA; [c] Vanderbilt School of Nursing, Nashville, TN, USA
* Corresponding author.
E-mail address: buffy.lupear@vanderbilt.edu

A primary focus for the modern health care agenda is to improve the quality and safety of patient care through the amelioration of adverse patient care events.[1,2] Improving the quality and safety of patient care is so valued; the Centers for Medicare and Medicaid Services (CMS) restricts the reimbursement of health care services based on the occurrence of adverse patient care events that they consider to be preventable, and should never occur.[3] One such adverse patient care event that the CMS has deemed should never occur is the development of a severe PU during a patient's admission to the hospital[3] (also known as a hospital-acquired PU [HAPU]).

CMS specifies a severe PU to be a stage III or stage IV PU.[3] Classification of a stage III and IV PU occurs when the tissue injury affects skin, muscle, bone, and conceivably tendons and joints.[4] Historically PUs have been associated with patients who have limited mobility, such as those confined to a bed or a wheelchair; and patients who are residents of long term care facilities, such as a nursing home or rehabilitation center. Along with this, previous thoughts were that the nurse/patient ratio, the acuity of the patient's health, and the educational level and experience of the nurse were also associated with the development of a PU.[5]

PROBLEM STATEMENT

Despite focused attention to improve the quality and safety of patient care, and the financial impact PUs can have on a health care provider or institution, evidence supports that PUs continue to occur in other patient populations during their admission to the hospital.[1] An example of a patient population in which evidence indicates that the development of PUs occurs is patients who have surgical procedures.[6]

The purpose of this project was to assess perioperative nurses' knowledge of risk factors considered indicators for PU development in the surgical patient population. The patient care area in which perioperative nurses practice is a single patient care entity referred to as the perioperative area. The perioperative area consists of three separate patient care areas: preoperative holding room (HR), operating room (OR), and postanesthesia care unit (PACU). Patients spend time in each of the 3 patient care areas during their admission to the perioperative area, with the exception of patients admitted directly to the OR from an intensive care unit or the emergency department.

Although nurse responsibilities are different in each of the patient care areas, there are some nurse responsibilities common to all 3 areas. The common nurse responsibilities may include patient assessments, effective communication during the transition of patient care from one patient care provider to another, and ensuring high quality and safe patient care during a patient's admission to the perioperative area. Therefore, it is necessary to assess the knowledge of all perioperative nurses relevant to indicators for PU development.

Technology Support for Project

The technology that supported this project was a Web-based survey system, Research Design and Capture (REDCap), and the hospital's e-mail system. A 10-minute survey was sent and returned via the Internet. REDCap allows validated data entry, audit trails to track data, and deidentification of data exported into statistical packages. REDCap is a known entity at the project site, assistance was readily available in using the application, and it was populated with the e-mail addresses of participants. Anonymity was ensured through the REDCap secure database and confidentiality was maintained.

BACKGROUND

More than 2 million people in the United States experience the effects of PUs each year.[7] Brem and colleagues[8] estimated that the cost to treat a stage IV PU averages $127,000 per patient, thereby contributing to the $11 billion financial impact that PUs generate on the US health care system. Of greater consequence are the 60,000 patients who die from the effects of PUs.[9] In understanding the cause of PUs, risk factors that are indicators for PU development, and the assessment tools currently used in identifying patients at risk, perioperative nurses have an opportunity to mitigate the development of PUs in the surgical patient population.

Cause of Pressure Ulcers

PUs result from an alteration in the integrity of skin and surrounding tissue. This alteration could be the product of decreased blood flow to the tissue or friction between the tissue and an external surface.[10]

Decreased blood flow

A decrease in blood flow to the tissue could be caused by prolonged pressure to the area of skin when a patient is stationary for an extended period, a severe decrease in the patient's body temperature, a significant and prolonged decrease in blood pressure, or an effect of a medication.

Friction

Patients with limited mobility do not have the capacity to move from one area to another without areas of their skin remaining in contact with an external surface. The external surface could be clothing, bed sheets, or a patient transfer device. When skin remains in contact with the external device during movement, friction occurs between the skin and the external surface. This friction can be diffuse and interrupt the integrity of the patient's skin, thereby enabling a PU to develop.

A challenge that health care providers encounter in the prevention of a PU is the limited ability to determine the exact time a PU develops. An example of this challenge is the failure to appreciate the severity of the initial insult to the underlying tissue until the external tissue shows signs of destruction.[1] As Walton-Greer[1] describes, tissue damage by appearance may not be evident for several hours to several days following surgery, thereby minimizing the association of PU development during a patient's admission to the perioperative area.

Pressure Ulcer Risk Assessment Tools

Since early in the 1960s, health care providers and researchers have struggled to create the perfect risk assessment tool to identify patients who are at risk for developing a PU.[11] The purpose of the tool is to prevent the development of a PU through early identification of those at risk. Each assessment tool has specific patient factors it considers risk factors for PU development. The overall score a patient receives on the assessment tool predicts the extent to which a patient is at risk for PU development.

Cubbin and Jackson

Created in 1991, The Cubbin and Jackson assessment tool has a validity of 89% sensitivity in predicting PU development, based on the scores of 10 patient metrics.[12(p200)] The metrics include weight, age, nutrition, mental capacity, vital signs, respiratory status, hygiene, and incontinence. The metric scores are 4 possible points with the overall highest score possible of 40 points. The lower the overall score, the higher the patient's risk for PU development.[12(p200)]

Douglas

The Douglas tool, developed in 1986, is a variation of the Norton assessment scale. With the highest sensitivity for predicting PU development (100%), the Douglas tool measures 7 patient metrics: activity, level of pain, nutrition, skin integrity, mental capacity, incontinence, and red blood cell volume.[12(p200)] The Douglas tool scores the patient metrics on either 3 or 4 points, with the highest possible score of 24 points. As with the Cubbin and Jackson tools, the higher the score, the lower the risk a patient has for developing a PU.[12(p200)]

Braden

According to Seongsook and colleagues[12] the Braden assessment tool is validated as having 97% sensitivity in predicting the development of a PU. The Braden tool, developed in 1987, determines a patient's risk for PU development based on 6 patient metrics: sensory function, moisture, activity, mobility, mechanical-shearing/friction, and nutrition. Similar to the Douglas tool, each metric is a 3-point or 4-point score, with the highest possible score of 23. A patient with a low Braden score (eg, 10) is at risk for developing a PU.[12(p200)]

Although these assessment tools have proved to be beneficial in certain patient populations, there is a question about the accuracy and sensitivity of the tools for risk of PU development in the surgical patient population. Evidence suggests that surgical, as well as patient, risk factors could serve as indicators that a surgical patient is at a higher risk for developing a PU.[6] This evidence limits the reliability for the risk assessments tools, such as the Braden, to serve as a sole indicator for PU development in the surgical patient population.[13]

PROJECT SIGNIFICANCE

As O'Brien and colleagues[6] identified, studies of PU development during a patient's admission to the perioperative area are limited. Despite a paucity of studies specific to the perioperative area, a significant percentage of PU development occurs in the surgical patient population.[6] In that the development of a PU in a surgical patient is an HAPU, the aim of this project was to identify potential knowledge deficits among perioperative nurses of indicators for PU development in the surgical patient population.

Effects of Pressure Ulcers

Health care

It is estimated that less than 5% of patients admitted to the hospital develop a PU; however, this percentage increases to more than 45% once the patient is admitted to the perioperative area.[14] Although this may not sound like a significant percentage, it is necessary to consider the number of surgical patients who are at risk for developing a PU in a medical center that admits more than 50,000 patients, and performs approximately 22,000 in-patient surgical procedures.[15] If 10% to 30% of these surgical patients develop a PU, then approximately 110 to 330 patients are at risk for developing a PU. Considering that the estimation for the cost of care for patients with PU is $127,000.00 per patient,[8] the resources necessary to care for this many patients ranges from $14 million to nearly $41.9 billion in health care costs.

Perioperative nursing

An estimated 80% of medical center admissions occur during the patients' admissions to the perioperative area on the day of their surgical procedures.[16] Therefore, perioperative nurses are often the initial health care providers for the surgical patient population as they prepare a patient for a surgical procedure. In that most PUs are preventable, perioperative nurses play a pivotal role in the prevention of PU development.

Advanced practice nursing

The roles and responsibilities of the advance practice nurse (APRN) are evolving with the changes in health care. With the increasing autonomy of practice, APRNs participate in the care of patients throughout a medical center, including the perioperative area. APRNs collaborate with perioperative nurses to ensure that surgical patients receive safe and high-quality care, thereby avoiding adverse events such as the development of a PU.

Patients

PUs not only create physical and emotional effects on the lives of patients and their families but financial effects as well.

Physical and emotional PUs cause patients to experience significant pain. Patients who develop a PU may require multiple hospital admissions and extensive surgical procedures to treat the PU. Scarring that occurs during the healing process of a PU can leave patients with a disfigured appearance. These physical effects of PUs can lead to surgical patients feeling isolated and depressed.

Financial Patients who develop PUs may require multiple hospital admissions and surgical procedures. These effects are not only emotionally and physically exhausting on a patient and family but they create a significant financial burden in health care costs and loss of wages.[8] O'Brien and colleagues[6] estimated the financial expenditure for health care of patients who developed a PU to range from $750 million to greater than $1 billion.

SYSTEM OF POPULATION IMPACT

In that a PU may begin at any point without obvious signs or symptoms, it is imperative for perioperative nurses to know and understand the risk factors that serve as indicators for potential PU development. Through knowledge and understanding of the indicators that predispose a surgical patient for developing a PU, perioperative nurses can take actions or perform interventions that mitigate the incidence of PUs developing.

The Institute for Healthcare Improvement contends that 2 undertakings must occur to prevent surgical patients from developing PUs: (1) identification of surgical patients with known indicators for PU development, and (2) implementation of appropriate interventions.[17] Types of interventions specific to surgical patients include, but are not limited to:

- Completion and documentation of thorough skin assessment by HR nurse, OR nurse, and PACU nurse
- Minimize skin's exposure to moisture
- Decrease incidence of sustained pressure to an area of skin
- Enhance optimal hydration
- Support temperature to maintain in the normal range

SYNTHESIS OF EVIDENCE

From October 2012 to May 2014, more than 200 articles pertaining to PUs were elicited from a MeSH search using the keywords and phrases "pressure ulcer" and "complication," and using the Boolean operator, "and." With the addition of the keywords "intraoperative," "perioperative," "postoperative," and "surgical," the literature search narrowed. Exclusion criteria consisted of literature not published in English and literature published more than 15 years ago. In addition to the exclusion criteria, evaluation of the articles occurred using the Preferred Reporting Items for Systematic Reviews and Meta-Analysis 2009 (PRISMA) checklist. By using this process, 8 articles were identified as specific to PU development in the perioperative area. These 8 articles consisted of literature reviews and quantitative studies. Identification of an additional 18 articles occurred through various Internet searches and article references.

A common theme was noted in the initial 8 articles; specific surgical procedure and patient factors were identified as indicators for PU development in surgical patients. Walton-Greer[1] offers a list of specific surgical procedure and patient factors that includes intraoperative patient temperature, length of surgical procedure, patient position required for surgery, hemoglobin and hematocrit levels, hemodynamic stability, preoperative albumin level, and comorbidities, such as diabetes mellitus (DM) and peripheral vascular disease (PVD).

Tschannen and colleagues[18] identified that the use of vasoactive medications to support a patient's blood pressure increased the incidence of PU development in the surgical patient by 33%. Tschannen and colleagues[18] also detailed that a surgical patient with the comorbidity of DM was 49% more likely to develop a PU than a patient without DM. With a 95% confidence interval, Scarletti and colleagues[19] acknowledged that a patient having a neurosurgical procedure was 3 times more likely to develop a PU than a patient presenting for a different procedure. Also recognized in this same study was that a patient receiving general anesthesia was 4.8 times more likely to develop a PU compared with a patient receiving local anesthesia.[19]

Although no study attests that a patient will definitely develop a PU by the mere fact of having a known indicator or exposure to an identified indictor, these studies do suggest that a surgical patient is at greater risk of developing a PU by having an identified indicator or exposure to an identified indicator.

There were 4 indicators apparent across the specific studies that should alert perioperative nurses that a surgical patient is at risk for developing a PU (**Box 1**).

Suggested limitations of studies relating to the development of PUs in surgical patients are inconsistent use of an electronic medical record and inaccurate documentation of the PU diagnosis code. Inconsistent and inaccurate documentation leads to an increased probability of missed data capture relative to PU development in patients who have had a surgical procedure. The potential for missed data capture implies that the incidence of PU development in the surgical patient population may be greater than was previously realized, thereby indentifying an opportunity for future research of PU development in the surgical patient population.

CONCEPTUAL AND THEORETIC MODELS

The initial conceptual model for this project focused broadly on perioperative-associated PU development. Although the initial concept highlighted factors associated with the development of a PU relative to each patient care area (the HR, the

---

Box 1
Four indicators that a patient is at risk for PU

1. Receiving vasoactive medications

2. Comorbidities

3. Type of surgical procedure

4. Type of anesthesia the patient receives.

OR, and the PACU), with time, the conceptual model transitioned to coincide with the nursing metaparadigm: nurse, person, environment, and health.[20] Through further iterations of this project, the conceptual model fully evolved to align with Myra Levine's[2] conservation model.

Levine Conservation Model

Myra Levine's[2] conservation model depicts the preservation of a patient's structural, personal, and social integrity, as well as energy through nursing care and by patients taking an active role in their care. The development of a PU in a surgical patient disrupts all 4 principles of the Levine[2] conservation model (**Box 2**).

Therefore, it is imperative for the perioperative nurses to maintain the patient's equilibrium between the principles of the Levine[2] conservation model and the patient's environment in order to preserve the surgical patients' structural, personal, and social integrity, as well as their energy.[2] This preservation can be accomplished through an appreciation and understanding of the indicators for PU development in surgical patients. Therefore, the knowledge and skills to assess patients at risk of PU development facilitates appropriate and earlier interventions by perioperative nurses.

PROJECT DESIGN
Project Setting

The facility that served as the project setting is a level I academic medical center. This medical center has 6 perioperative areas, and, of these 6 areas, 1 specific perioperative area was the practice setting for this project. This perioperative area consists of 25 individual HRs, 11 ORs, and a 14-bay PACU. The typical patient population includes current in-patients, patients scheduled to go home following surgery, patients admitted to the hospital on the day of their surgery, and patients admitted for a 23-hour observation following surgery. This setting correlates well with this project design with its variety of surgical procedures, patient population, and consistent nursing staff.

Participants: Perioperative Nurses

Following approval of the institution's internal review board, communication was made with the nursing leadership to explain the purpose, intention, and potential benefits of this project. All perioperative nurses in the specific area chosen were eligible and encouraged to participate in an assessment survey. The perioperative nurses included in this project practice in one of 3 patient care areas within a larger perioperative entity.

Box 2
Four principles disrupted by PU in a surgical patient

- Structural integrity: an interruption in tissue and muscle integrity.

- Energy: increased requirements necessary for healing, leaving a patient unable to perform activities of daily living. Evidence suggests that PUs create an inflammatory response by the body, consequently increasing the energy expenditure and resulting in anorexia and loss of important nutrients.[27]

- Personal integrity: effects of PU scarring and threat of financial instability caused by inability to work.

- Social integrity: feelings of isolation caused by hospitalizations and separation from loved ones.

Holding room nurse
The HR nurse prepares patients for their surgical procedures.

Operating room nurse
The OR nurse provides support for the patient, OR team, and surgeon during a surgical procedure.

Postanesthesia care unit nurse
The PACU nurse assesses and monitors the surgical patient's vital signs after the patient has received an anesthetic for a surgical procedure.

Each perioperative area has established nurse responsibilities for patient care, as detailed in **Box 3**. Common nurse responsibilities shared in each of the 3 patient care areas, with the overall common responsibility of providing safe and high-quality patient care, are shown in **Table 1**. Examples of common responsibilities in each patient care area include the appropriate identification of the surgical patient; performing, as well as documenting, a patient assessment inclusive of skin assessments; and review of the patient's medical history.

The perioperative area used in this project uses approximately 50 perioperative nurses who are registered nurses (RNs) with varied levels of clinical experience and educational background. In that this medical center has obtained Magnet recognition, an overall focus of the institution is supportive of all RNs completing their bachelor of science in nursing (BSN). Historically, for an RN, the years and type of clinical experience were valued as more important than the amount and type of education. However, evidence indicates that hospitals that use RNs with a minimum of a BSN degree have lower incidences of adverse patient outcomes.[21]

This select area has perioperative nurses with years of experience ranging from recent nursing graduates to nurses who have been practicing for more than 20 years. Although these specific perioperative nurses may have many years of clinical practice experience, they may only have a few years of clinical experience in the perioperative area. Despite the differences in the level of experience, or education, all nurses in this perioperative area are RNs.

Assessing Perioperative Nurses' Knowledge

Having the appropriate information is essential before making an operational decision.[22] A common misconception is that an assessment and an evaluation achieve the same goals.[22] As Krau and Maxwell[23] describe, the information obtained through an assessment directs the next steps of action needed. Different from the information gathered through an assessment, the information gathered through an evaluation provides the feedback necessary to determine whether an objective was accomplished.[23]

Fifty-two perioperative nurses received a link to a 16-question assessment tool, in the form of a survey, via e-mail. The content of the questions assessed the perioperative nurses' knowledge of 4 indicators identified in the literature to be relevant to the development of a PU and to align with the Levine[2] conservation model: structural-physiologic indicators, energy-surgical indicators, personal-assessment indicators, and social-communication indicators.

Physiologic
Comorbidities, abnormal laboratory values, hemodynamic stability, and the patient's intraoperative temperature; as well as the perioperative nurses' level of education, primary area of practice, and PU education.

Box 3
Responsibilities of perioperative nurses

Perioperative nurses' patient care responsibilities by area

Holding Room (HR)

  Perform a patient history and full patient assessment including a full skin assessment

  Start patient's intravenous access

  Confirm surgical procedure, surgeon, and surgical site

  Ensure preoperative surgical and anesthesia orders are complete

  Ensure surgical consent is available and complete

  Perform a patient care handover with in-room anesthesia provider

  Complete required preoperative documentation

Operating Room (OR)

  Identify surgical patient, review patient history, and assess surgical patient

  Confirm surgical procedure, surgical site, surgeon, and surgical consent is complete

  Ensure the sterility and availability of surgical instruments

  Maintains accurate count of surgical instruments before the beginning and at the conclusion of surgical procedure

  Confirms patient position required and necessary positioning devices for surgical procedure

  Assists with movement and positioning of surgical patient

  Completes required intraoperative documentation

Postanesthesia care unit (PACU)

  Reviews patient medical history and surgical procedure with in-room anesthesia provider and OR registered nurse (RN)

  Perform a full patient assessment, including a full skin assessment

  Monitor patient's postanesthesia vital signs

  Ensure postoperative surgical and anesthesia orders are complete

  Complete required postanesthesia documentation

Surgical
Length of surgery, position required for surgery, and type of anesthesia required; as well as the restrictions placed on the patient during the healing process (eg, limited motion).

Assessment
Skin assessment tools were available and used (eg, Braden, Cubbin and Jackson, the Douglas scale); as well as the emotional struggles patients with PUs may experience and the perioperative nurses' perspective based on experience.

Communication
Current processes in place for the transfer of patient care information between the perioperative patient care areas, as well as the isolation patients may experience because of long hospitalizations.

Data Collection Tool

The collection of the assessment data occurred through a research electronic data capturing system (REDCap) that facilitates the electronic collection and secure

Table 1
Comparison of perioperative nurses' patient care responsibilities

Patient Care Responsibility	HR	OR	PACU
Patient identification/verification per hospital policy	X	X	X
Obtains/reviews patient's medical history	X	X	X
Performs patient skin assessment	X	X	X
Confirms surgical procedure, site, surgeon, and consent	X	X	—
Ensures preoperative surgical and anesthesia orders are complete	X	—	—
Performs patient care handover during transition of care between perioperative areas	X	X	X
Completes required documentation for specific perioperative area	X	X	X
Ensures the sterility and availability of surgical instruments	—	X	—
Confirms position of patient for surgical procedure	—	X	—
Ensures intraoperative surgical and anesthesia orders are complete	—	X	—
Maintains accurate count of surgical equipment before and at the conclusion of the surgical procedure	—	X	—
Assists with the movement and positioning of patient for surgical procedure	—	X	—
Monitors the patient's postanesthesia vital signs	—	—	X
Ensures postoperative surgical and anesthesia orders are complete	—	—	X

storage of data, thereby allowing the data to be readily available for use in research endeavors.[24] REDCap is an intuitive system allowing a person to develop an electronic assessment tool with ease, and minimizes the need for additional support staff. Technology advances have improved the ease with which research via surveys may occur, be gathered, analyzed, and categorized, and assists data collection to adhere to multiple stop gaps for participant confidentiality and security of data.

The design of the functions of REDCap ensures that the captured data are deidentified, credible, and valid for analysis. The REDCap system required questions to be structured in a specific manner, and allowed questions to have branching logic and the developer to stipulate when a question was required to be answered before the survey submission.[24]

The data collection tool (**Fig. 1**) used in this project consisted of 16 questions assessing the perioperative nurses' baseline knowledge of indicators for PU development in the surgical patient population, previous education relative to PU development, and other demographic information. It was important when developing the questions to assess the perioperative nurses' level of knowledge, not their ability to guess an answer.[25] Therefore, wording of the questions and possible responses were consistent in content, tense, and grammar.

DATA ANALYSIS AND RESULTS

As a nonexperimental study of a single group of participants with 2 or more variables measured for each participant, an Excel spreadsheet was used to capture the

Perioperative Nursing Assessment Tool

Hello-

A focus of attention in today’s healthcare environment is on improvement of quality and safety of patient care. One such improvement is through the prevention of adverse patient-care events such as the development of a pressure ulcer (PU). Pressure Ulcers that develop during a patient’s hospital admission are called hospital-acquired pressure ulcers (HAPU). Although much attention is on the prevention of patients developing Hospital Acquired Pressure Ulcers, evidence demonstrates this adverse patient-care event continues to occur.

The following is a short 12-question survey to assess perioperative nurses' knowledge of risk factors for the development of Hospital Acquired Pressure Ulcers in patients. Completion of this survey will take approximately 5-10 minutes of your time, and is strictly voluntary. By completing this survey, you acknowledge informed consent for the use of this anonymous and de-identified information to develop quality improvement initiatives.

◆

Thank you for your time and participation,

Buffy Krauser Lupear

615-936-2728

The following are multiple-choice questions. Please select the correct answer.

The following surgical procedure is associated with a three times higher incidence of patient developing a hospital acquired pressure ulcer.	☐ Hepatobiliary ☐ Orthopedic ☐ Neurosurgery ☐ Otolaryngology (Please select the correct answer)
The following lab value is an indicator a surgical patient is at higher risk for developing a hospital acquired pressure ulcer.	☐ Hemoglobin (Hgb) AlC of 5 mg/dL (normal value < 5.7%) ☐ Hematocrit of 43% (normal value male 40.7-50.3%; normal female 36.1-44.3%) ☐ Albumin of 2.9g/dL (normal value 3.4-5.4 g/dL) ☐ Blood Urea Nitrogen (BUN) of 22mg/dL (normal value 6-20mg/dL) ☐ None of the Above (Please select the correct answer)
The preoperative, intra-operative, or post-operative use of which medications increases the chance of a patient developing a hospital acquired pressure ulcer.	☐ Nitroglycerin, Metoprolol ☐ Phenylephrine, Ephedrine ☐ Metoprolol, Phenylephrine ☐ Ephedrine, Nitroglycerin (Please select the correct answer)

Fig. 1. REDCap survey.

downloaded data from REDCap for analysis. In correlation with the Levine[2] conservation model, the data identified the perioperative nurses':

- Structural integrity: baseline knowledge of the physiologic factors for PU development
- Energy: understanding of the surgical factors that affect the development of PUs
- Personal integrity: perceptions of the emotions experienced by patients who have developed PUs
- Social integrity: perceptions of perioperative communications during the transfer of patient care between perioperative areas and the awareness of when a surgical patient does develop a PU

Fifty-two perioperative nurses received a link to the REDCap survey. At the end of the 2-week period, 23 perioperative nurses participated, completed, and submitted the survey; a participation response rate of 44%.

The following medical condition is an indicator that a surgical patient is at higher risk for developing a hospital acquired pressure ulcer.	☐ Cirrhosis of the Liver ☐ Pancreatitis ☐ End Stage Renal Disease ☐ Diabetes Mellitus (Please select the correct answer)
The incidence of hospital acquired pressure ulcer development is decreased when...	☐ The surgical procedure is 6 hours and the patient is padded appropriately ☐ The patient has multiple surgical procedures in an effort to keep all procedures 6 hours or less ☐ The patient's surgical procedure is 6 hours with local anesthesia and sedation only ☐ The surgical procedure is 6 hours and the patient's temperature is maintained at 36 degrees Celsius (Please select the correct answer)
The development of a hospital acquired pressure ulcer affects the surgical patient by...	☐ Allowing patients to play an active role in his/her health care decisions ☐ Limiting the patient's ability to perform basic activities of daily living ☐ Enhancing the patient's body composition and appearance through organized physical rehabilitation (Please select the correct answer)
What is the impact of hospital acquired pressure ulcers on a patient's metabolic requirements and expenditure?	☐ A hospital acquired pressure ulcer increases a patient's metabolic requirements and expenditures due to an inflammatory response in the body ☐ A hospital acquired pressure ulcer decreases a patient's metabolic requirement/expenditure due to his/her decreased mobility ☐ A hospital acquired pressure ulcer does not affect a patient's metabolic requirement/expenditure as long as the patient does not have an associated fever (Please select the correct answer)

Answer the Following Question Based on your Perspective as a Perioperative Nurse

When a patient develops a hospital acquired pressure ulcer, the patient experiences many emotions. From your perspective as a perioperative nurse please list what you believe are three major emotions experienced by a patient who develops a hospital acquired pressure ulcer:	☐(Please list your 3 answers)

Please Indicate the Answer that Best Reflects Your Experience and Perspective as a Perioperative Nurse

The initial physiological insult leading to the development of hospital acquired pressure ulcers occurs infrequently in the perioperative area when compared to other patient care units.	☐ Strongly Disagree ☐ Disagree ☐ Agree ☐ Strongly Agree
Perioperative nurses can influence the development of a hospital acquired pressure ulcer.	☐ Strongly Disagree ☐ Disagree ☐ Agree ☐ Strongly Agree

Fig. 1. (*continued*).

Structural Integrity and Energy

In order for perioperative nurses to maintain the structural integrity of the patient, as well as have influence on the energy aspect of the Levine[2] conservation model, it is essential for perioperative nurses to know and understand the physiologic and surgical factors that affect the development of a PU. To appreciate the perioperative nurses' knowledge of PUs it was necessary to assess the perioperative nurses' baseline knowledge, highest level of nursing education, years of nursing experience, primary area of perioperative nursing practice, previous PU education, and years since PU education.

Baseline knowledge of pressure ulcer indicators

The information obtained from the survey resulted in a variety of responses concerning the participants' knowledge. Although no single question had 100% of the participants answer correctly, 4 of the 7 knowledge questions had greater than 60% of the participants provide correct answers (**Table 2**). In contrast, all participants incorrectly answered question 2 concerning specific laboratory values associated with PU development.

During the transition of care between the perioperative areas, perioperative nurses report the factors that influence the likelihood of a patient developing a hospital acquired pressure ulcers.

☐ Strongly Disagree
☐ Disagree
☐ Agree
☐ Strongly Agree

The perioperative nurse is notified if a patient develops a hospital acquired pressure ulcer after the patient has been discharged from the perioperative area.

☐ Strongly Disagree
☐ Disagree
☐ Agree
☐ Strongly Agree

Demographics

What is your highest level of nursing education?

☐ Diploma
☐ Associate Degree
☐ Bachelor of Science in Nursing
☐ Masters of Science in Nursing
☐ Doctorate of Nursing Practice
☐ Doctorate of Philosophy
☐ Other: _____

Please indicate your level of nursing education.

_____

How many years of experience do you have as a nurse?

☐ 0-5
☐ 6-10
☐ 11-15
☐ >16

What are your total years of experience as a perioperative nurse?

☐ 0-5
☐ 6-10
☐ 11-15
☐ >16

Where is your primary area of perioperative nursing practice at Vanderbilt University Medical Center?

☐ Holding Room
☐ Operating Room
☐ Post Anesthesia Care Unit (PACU)

Where have you received information or education regarding hospital acquired pressure ulcer development??

☐ Work sponsored in-service
☐ Nursing Conference
☐ Nursing Education Curriculum
☐ Journal Article
☐ Online in-service/webinar
☐ Have not received education regarding Hospital Acquired Pressure Ulcers
☐ Other_____

Please indicate where you have received information or education on the development of hospital acquired pressure ulcers.

_____

How many years since has it been since you received any information or education on the development of hospital acquired pressure ulcers?

☐ < 1
☐ 2-4
☐ >5
☐ N/A

Fig. 1. (*continued*).

Highest level of nursing education

The percentage of perioperative nurses who have a diploma or associate degree is slightly higher than the percentage of nurses who have a BSN. degree; 48% compared with 44%. An additional 8% have an MSN or other master's degree. None of the perioperative nurses has a degree higher than master's level (**Fig. 2**).

Years of nursing experience

Fig. 3 shows that 83% of perioperative nurses have 11 years or more of nursing experience, with 74% having greater than 16 years of experience. Of the 83% with 11 or more years of experience, less than 45% have similar years of experience as a perioperative nurse. Fifty-six percent of participant perioperative nurses have 10 years or less perioperative nursing experience.

Primary site of perioperative nursing practice

Of the 52 invitations sent, 6 of the nurses primarily work in the OR setting, with the remaining working in the HR and PACU settings. **Fig. 4** shows the percentage participation of RNs from each area. The HR setting yielded the highest participation of nurses at 39%, with the OR participation at 35%.

Pressure ulcer education

Ninety-one percent of perioperative nurse participants acknowledged having a form of PU education, most either during a work-sponsored in-service or during their

Table 2
Perioperative nurses' assessment: baseline knowledge

Perioperative Nurses' Assessment of Indicators for PU Development in Surgical Patient Populations

Question	Option 1	Option 2	Option 3	Option 4	Option 5
The following surgical procedure is associated with a 3 times higher incidence of patient developing a hospital-acquired PU	Hepatobiliary 17.4%	Orthopedic 56.5%	ªNeurosurgery 21.7%	Otolaryngology 4.3%	None of the above
n	4	13	5	1	
The following laboratory values indicate that a surgical patient is at higher risk for developing an HAPU	Hemoglobin A1c level of 5 mg/dL 13.0%	ªAlbumin level of 2.9 g/dL 0.0%	Hematocrit level of 43% 52.2%	BUN level of 22 mg/dL 8.7%	None of the above 26.1%
n	3	0	12	2	6
The preoperative, intraoperative or postoperative use of which medications increases the chance of a patient developing an HAPU	Nitroglycerin, metoprolol 21.7%	ªPhenylephrine, ephedrine 65.2%	Metoprolol, phenylephrine 4.3%	Ephedrine, nitroglycerin 8.7%	
n	5	15	1	2	
The following medical condition is an indicator that a surgical patient is at higher risk for developing an HAPU	Cirrhosis of the liver 8.7%	Pancreatitis 0.0%	End-stage renal disease 8.7%	ªDM 82.6%	

n	2	0	2	19

The incidence of HAPU development is decreased when....	The surgical procedure is 6 h and the patient is padded appropriately	The patient has multiple surgical procedures in an effort to keep all procedures 6 h or less	[a] The patient's surgical procedure is 6 h with local anesthesia and sedation only	The surgical procedure is 6 h and the patient's temperature is maintained at 36°
	43.5%	17.4%	8.7%	30.4%
n	10	4	2	7

The development of an HAPU affects the surgical patient by....	Allowing patients to play an active role in their health care decisions	[a] Limiting the patient's ability to perform basic activities of daily living	Enhancing the patient's body composition and appearance through organized physical rehabilitation	—
	4.3%	95.7%	0.0%	—
n	1	22	0	—

What is the impact of HAPUs on a patient's metabolic requirements and expenditure?	[a] An HAPU increases a patient's metabolic requirements and expenditures because of an inflammatory response in the body	An HAPU decreases a patient's metabolic requirement/expenditure because of decreased mobility	An HAPU does not affect a patient's metabolic requirement/expenditure as long as the patient does not have an associated fever	—
	95.7%	4.3%	0.0%	—
n	22	1	0	—

Total participants: n = 23.
Abbreviation: BUN, blood urea nitrogen.
[a] Denotes correct answer.

Chart Title

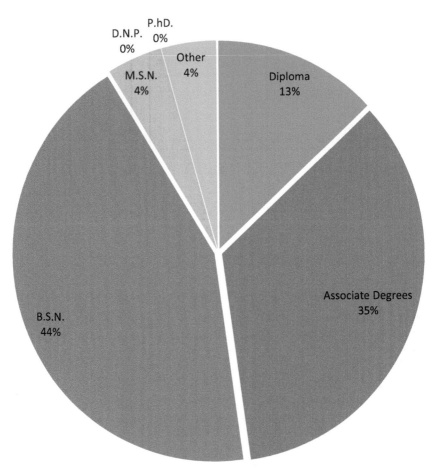

Fig. 2. Highest level of RNs' nursing education. BSN, bachelor of science in nursing; DNP, doctorate of nursing practice; MSN, master of science in nursing.

nursing curriculum. Eight percent of the perioperative nurses who completed the survey have 5 years or less of nursing experience, which could indicate that some have not had PU education since nursing school. Alarmingly, 9% of the participants who responded indicated that they have not had education related to PUs (**Fig. 5**).

Years since pressure ulcer education

Approximately 78% of the participants have had some form of PU education in the past 4 years (**Fig. 6**). Twenty-one percent indicated a greater than 5-year period since such an educational opportunity, or that no such education occurred.

Personal and Social Integrity

The personal and social integrity aspect of the Levine[2] model was important in understanding how the perioperative nurses perceived that the patient would respond

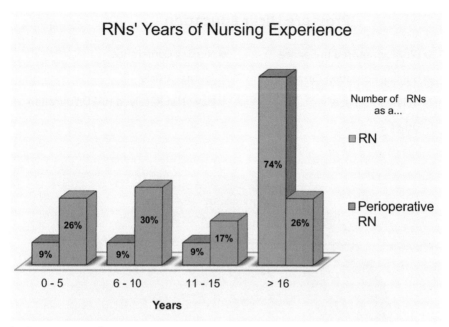

Fig. 3. RNs' years of nursing experience.

emotionally to developing a PU, as well as the perioperative nurses' perception regarding communication during the transition of patient care. It was equally important to appreciate whether the perioperative nurses comprehended that PUs could begin in the perioperative area, and that they could influence the development of PUs.

Perceived emotional response to pressure ulcer development by patients
The survey offered an opportunity for the participants to list 3 emotional responses they perceived patients who developed a PU would experience. Although there was

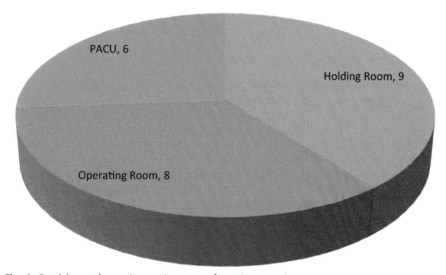

Fig. 4. Participants by perioperative area of nursing practice.

Pressure Ulcer Education

- Work Sponsored In-Service
- Nursing Conference
- Nursing Education Cirrculum
- Journal Article
- Online In-service/Webinar
- Have Not Received HAPU Education
- Other

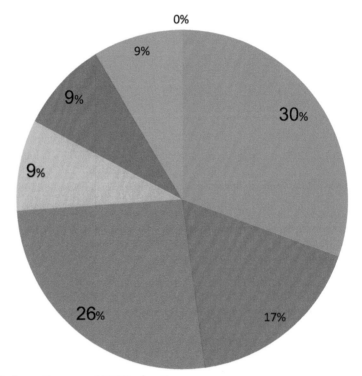

Fig. 5. Perioperative nurses' HAPU education.

a potential for 69 possible responses, the total number of responses listed on the survey by the participants was 64. The responses were grouped into 15 categories: anger, depression, frustration, fear, pain, anxiety, helplessness, body image, embarrassment, disappointment, disbelief, apathy, burden, monetary, and other (**Fig. 7**). Most of the emotions the participants perceived that patients experienced were in the anger, depression, and frustration categories. Relative to the Levine[2] conservation model, these results support that PUs interrupt a patient's personal and social integrity, thereby indicating the import role that perioperative nurses have in preventing the development of PUs in surgical patients.

Perspective based on registered nurse experience

The survey prompted the participants to describe their perspectives of communication and the impact that perioperative nurses have concerning PU development. As noted in **Table 3**, most perioperative nurses agreed, or strongly agreed, that

Most Recent HAPU Education

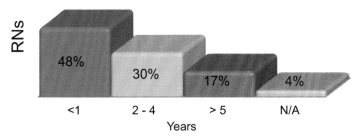

Fig. 6. Most recent HAPU education. N/A, not available.

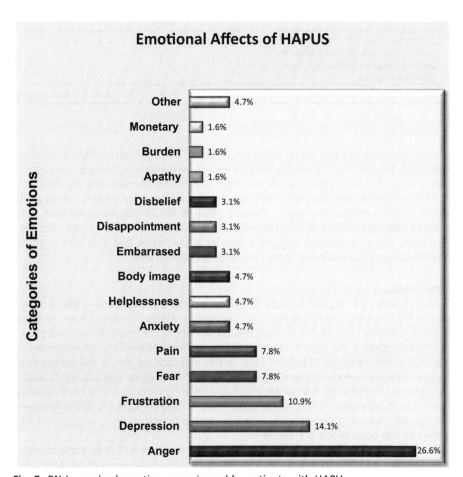

Fig. 7. RNs' perceived emotions experienced by patients with HAPUs.

Table 3
Perioperative nurses' perspective

Perioperative Nurses' Assessment: Perspective and Experience As a Perioperative Nurse				
	Strongly Disagree (%)	Disagree (%)	Agree (%)	Strongly Agree (%)
The initial physiologic insult leading to the development of HAPUs occurs infrequently in the perioperative area compared with other patient care units	8.7	52.2	34.8	4.3
n	2	12	8	1
Perioperative nurses can influence the development of an HAPU	4.3	4.3	39.1	52.2
n	1	1	9	12
During the transition of care between the perioperative areas, perioperative nurses report the factors that influence the likelihood of a patient developing an HAPU	8.7	47.8	39.1	4.3
n	2	11	9	1
The perioperative nurse is notified if a patient develops an HAPU after the patient has been discharged from the perioperative area	52.2	39.1	8.7	0.0
n	12	9	2	0

Total participants: n = 23.

perioperative nurses have the ability to influence the development of PUs. On further evaluation, **Fig.** 8A and B illustrate the diversity of perceptions specific to the perioperative area of nursing practice. For example, 75% of HR nurses strongly disagree, and 75% of OR nurses disagree, that the initial physiologic insult of a PU infrequently occurs in the perioperative area, whereas 50% of PACU nurses agree and 50% disagree that the initial insult for PU development infrequently occurs in the perioperative area. These responses suggest a lack of appreciation that PUs can begin to develop during a patient's admission to the perioperative area.

Communication
The participants also agreed regarding notification that a perioperative patient developed a PU following discharge from the perioperative area. **Table 3** shows findings that 39% disagree, and 52.2% strongly disagree, that this communication takes place. Slightly less clear is the communication of factors that influence the development of PUs during the transition of patient care. In this instance, 47.8% of the participants disagree that this communication occurs, whereas 39.1% agree that the communication does occur. Similarly, the participants have differing perceptions of the frequency with which PUs develop in the perioperative area. As noted in **Table 3**, 52.2% disagree that the adverse event occurs infrequently in the perioperative area, whereas 34.8% agree that the occurrence is infrequent.

The transition of care is a critical point for the communication of patient information, or in this case lack of communication. As previously mentioned, separation of the data into specific work area groups occurred, with the responses being scattered

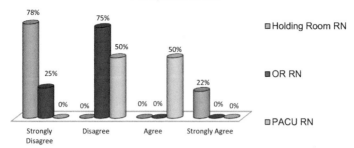

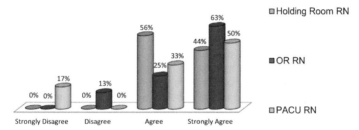

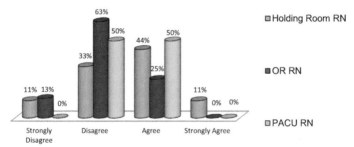

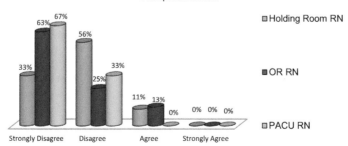

Fig. 8. Perioperative nurse's perspectives by area of practice. (*A*) Physiologic insult. (*B*) RN influence. (*C*) Transition of care. (*D*) Follow up.

throughout a spectrum of responses (see **Fig. 8C**). This finding is exemplified by the participants' responses of strongly disagreeing, disagreeing, agreeing, or strongly agreeing to the following statement: "During the transition of care between perioperative areas, perioperative nurses report factors that influence the likelihood of a patient developing an HAPU." Fifty percent of the PACU nurses agreed and 50% disagreed that this communication occurred. The HR nurses' responses were similar, in which 44% agreed and 33% disagreed. None of the perioperative areas had more than 55% of the participants agree or strongly agree that communication of this information occurs. **Fig. 8D** provides the perspective of the perioperative nurses related to awareness of whether a surgical patient did develop a PU following discharge from the perioperative area. Overwhelmingly, a collective 64% of the nurses disagree and strongly disagree that any notification occurs.

PROJECT SUMMARY

Understanding the origins of nursing conceptual models encompasses the nursing metaparadigm; as previously acknowledged, the conceptual models of nursing have a binding relationship with clinical practice.[20,26] Supported by the concepts of the Levine[2] conservation model the aim of this project was to identify areas that are in need of improvement to ensure that the surgical patient population receives high-quality and safe patient care, and to ameliorate the adverse event of a surgical patient developing a PU.

Perioperative nurses have a critical opportunity to preserve surgical patients' personal, social, and structural integrity, as well as their energy.[2] However, they must have the tools and knowledge to do so. The data obtained from this survey met the objective and purpose of this project by assessing the perioperative nurses' knowledge relative to the indicators for PU development in the surgical patient population. The overall findings suggest the need for evidence-based PU education and opportunities to improve communication during the transition of care from one perioperative area to another.

Impact of Project Results on Practice

The information gained through the survey has highlighted more than 1 opportunity to improve patient care and eventual outcomes. Although the survey contained 7 questions related to the cause and indicators for PU development, the responses varied. Despite a 44% participation rate of the perioperative nurses, the variation in responses indicates that the perioperative nurses do not have full understanding and knowledge of the evidence-based indicators for PU development. Providing perioperative nurses with evidence-based education about the indicators for PU development is essential to ensure high-quality and safe care for surgical patients.

The data also point out inconsistencies in the patient workflow process during the transition of patient care. The indication of incomplete or inconsistent communication during the transition of patient care suggests that opportunities for adverse patient outcomes are present. Incorporating patient-specific and surgical procedure–specific indicators that place surgical patients at risk for developing a PU is essential to ensure the prevention of PU development.

Strengths and Limitations of Project

This project highlighted that the development of a PU may begin at any point during a patient's admission to the hospital. The benefits of PU prevention are not merely 1-sided; PUs affect everyone in the health care industry, especially the patients.

Strengths

An important strength of this project was bringing awareness of the problem to those who can influence it the most. Speaking with the perioperative nurses revealed that most did not give much thought to PUs, because they did not appreciate the ambiguity associated with the inability to pinpoint the exact time a PU begins to develop. An additional strength of this project was rekindling the eagerness of perioperative nurses to learn something new and different. Immediately following the release of the survey, perioperative nurses were asking for the answers and explanations to the questions related to the indicators of PU development. Answers to survey questions were not given to the participants during the project data collection time so as to not influence the responses.

The most important strength is in the identification of evidence-based surgical and patient factors that serve as indicators for PU development in the surgical patient population. Just as important is the appreciation of the impact that PUs have on patients' structural, personal, and social integrity, as well as their energy. The Levine[2] conservation model eloquently depicts the delicate balance between patient and environment that perioperative nurses must maintain to promote surgical patients' structural, personal, and social integrity, as well as the patients' energy. In maintaining the Levine[2] conservation model, perioperative nurses ensure that surgical patients receive safe and high-quality patient care.

Limitations

Despite the eagerness of perioperative nurses to participate in the survey, the overall participation was approximately 44%. The small sample size (23 participants) leaves room to question whether the results were a true reflection of perioperative nurses' knowledge of indicators for PU development in the surgical patient population. Several perioperative nurses alluded to the difficulty of the questions, and thought that they did not know the answers; therefore, they were reluctant to complete the survey.

SUMMARY

It is essential that nurses have the information and tools necessary to meet the needs of patients and society. Evidence identified during this project dispels the historical assumptions that preventing PUs is not possible. This evidence provides specific knowledge that can facilitate appropriate nursing actions, thereby enabling perioperative nurses to take an active role in the prevention of PUs in the surgical patient population. This project has highlighted the need to bring awareness of evidence-based indicators for PU development to all of the perioperative areas within the practice setting. Technology has improved the day-to-day availability education in the workplace and may be the route (online education modules) for dissemination of information to improve patient care.

The findings of this project suggest a gap in the evidence-based knowledge of perioperative nurses for indicators of PU development in the surgical patient population. An unintended finding of this project was a need to improve patient workflow processes during the transition of patient care from one perioperative area to another.

The findings of this project, through literature review and assessing the perioperative nurses' knowledge, allow the development of PU assessment tools and evidence-based PU education specific to the surgical patient population. Only with knowledge and tools specific for PU development in the surgical patient population can perioperative nurses mitigate the incidence of PU development during surgical patients' admission to the perioperative area.

REFERENCES

1. Walton-Greer P. Prevention of pressure ulcers in the surgical patient. AORN J 2009;89(3):538–48.
2. Levine ME. The four conservation principles of nursing. Nurs Forum 1967;6(1): 45–59. Available at: http://onlinelibrary.wiley.com.proxy.library.vanderbilt.edu/ doi/10.1111/j.1744-6198.1967.tb01297.x/pdf.
3. Medicare takes new steps to make your hospital stay safer. In: Centers for Medicare and Medicaid Services. 2008. Available at: http://cms.gov/Newsroom/ MediaReleaseDatabase/Fact-Sheet/2008. Accessed September 28, 2013.
4. National Pressure Ulcer Advisory Panel. 2014. Available at: http://www. npuap.org/resources/educational-and-clinical-resources/npuap-pressure-ulcer-stagescategories/. Accessed January 16, 2014.
5. Wurster J. What role can nurse leaders play in reducing the incidence of pressure sores? Nurs Econ 2007;25(5):267–9. Available at: http://www.medscape.com/ viewarticle/565606_4.
6. O'Brien D, Shanks A, Talsma A, et al. Intraoperative risk factors associated with postoperative pressure ulcers in critically ill patients: a retrospective observational study. Crit Care Med 2013;41(11):1–7. http://dx.doi.org/10.1097/CCM. 0b013e318298a849.
7. Young D, Shen J, Estocado N, et al. Financial impact of improved pressure ulcer staging in the acute hospital with use of a new tool, the NE1 Wound Assessment Tool. Adv Skin Wound Care 2012;25(4):158–66.
8. Brem H, Maggi J, Nierman D, et al. High cost of stage IV pressure ulcers. Am J Surg Pathol 2010;200(4):473–7. http://dx.doi.org/10.1016/j.amjsurg. 2009.12.021.
9. Fred C, Ford S, Wagner D, et al. Intraoperatively acquired pressure ulcers and perioperative normothermia: a look at relationships. AORN J 2012;96(3): 251–60. http://dx.doi.org/10.1016/j.aorn.2012.06.014.
10. Bouten CV, Oomens CW, Baaijens FP, et al. The etiology of pressure ulcers: skin deep or muscle. Arch Phys Med Rehabil 2003;84:616–9. http://dx.doi.org/10. 1053/apmr.2003.50038.
11. Lindgren M, Unosson M, Krantz A, et al. A risk assessment scale for the prediction of pressure sore development: reliability and validity. J Adv Nurs 2002;38(2):190–9. Available at: www.wirral.nhs.uk/uploads/document/ RsikassesscakeforPSstudy.pdf.
12. Seongsook J, Ihnsook J, Younghee L. Validity of pressure ulcer risk assessment scales: Cubbin and Jackson, Braden, and Douglas scale. Int J Nurs Stud 2003; 41(2004):199–204. http://dx.doi.org/10.1016/S0020-7489(03)00135-4.
13. Hyun S, Vermillion B, Newton C, et al. Predictive validity of the Braden scale for patients in the intensive care units. Am J Crit Care 2013;22(6):514–20.
14. Price MC, Whitney JD, King CA. Development of a risk assessment tool for intraoperative pressure ulcers. J Wound Ostomy Continence Nurs 2005;32(1):19–30.
15. US News and World Report. 2014. Available at: http://health.usnews.com/best-hospitals/area/tn/vanderbilt-university-medical-center-6521060.   Accessed October 10, 2013.
16. Sullivan ES. Skin assessment and prevention of pressure ulcers: the role of the perianesthesia nurse. J Perianesth Nurs 2008;23(4):262–4. http://dx.doi.org/10. 1016/j.jopan.2008.05.2004.
17. Pressure ulcers. In: Pressure ulcers. 2013. Available at: http://www.ihi.org/ explore/PressureUlcers/Page/default. Accessed January 17, 2014.

18. Tschannen D, Bates O, Talsma A, et al. Patient-specific and surgical characteristics in the development of pressure ulcers. Am J Crit Care 2012;21(2):116–24.
19. Scarletti KC, Michel JL, Gamba MA, et al. Pressure ulcers in surgery patients: incidence and associated factors. Rev Esc Enferm USP 2011;45(6):1369–75. Available at: www.ee.usp.br/reeusp/.
20. Chinn P, Kramer M. Integrated theory and knowledge development in nursing. 8th edition. St Louis (MO): Elsevier Mosby; 2011.
21. Aiken LH, Clarke SP, Cheung RB, et al. Educational levels of hospital nurses and surgical patient mortality. J Am Med Assoc 2003;290(12):1617–23. Available at: http://jama.jamanetwork.com/.
22. Watkins R, Guerra IJ. How do you determine whether assessment or evaluation is required. ASTD T & OD Sourcebook; 2002. p. 131–9. Available at: http://home.gwu.edu/~rwatkins/articles/howdoyou.pdf.
23. Krau SD, Maxwell CA. Creating a tool to evaluate patient performance. Nurs Clin North Am 2011;46:351–65. http://dx.doi.org/10.1016/j.cnur.2011.05.009.
24. Harris PA, Taylor R, Thielke R, et al. Research electronic data capture (REDCap) –A metadata-driven methodology and workflow process for providing translational research informatics support. J Biomed Inform 2009;42(2):377–81.
25. Su WM, Osisek PJ, Montgomery C, et al. Designing multiple choice test items at higher cognitive levels. Nurse Educ 2009;34(5):223–7. Available at: https://ovidsp.tx.ovid.com.proxy.library.vanderbilt.edu.
26. Fawcett J. Conceptual models and nursing practice: the reciprocal relationship. J Adv Nurs 1992;17:224–8. Available at: http://onlinelibrary.wiley.com.proxy.library.vanderbilt.edu/doi/10.1111/j.1365-2648.1992.tb01877.x/pdf.
27. Cereda E, Klersy C, Rondanelli M, et al. Energy balance in patients with pressure ulcers: a systematic review and meta-analysis of observational studies. J Am Diet Assoc 2011;111(12):1868–76. http://dx.doi.org/10.1016/j.jada.2011.09.005.

Index

Note: Page numbers of article titles are in **boldface** type.

http://dx.doi.org/10.1016/S0029-6465(15)00038-9
0029-6465/15/$ – see front matter © 2015 Elsevier Inc. All rights reserved.
nursing.theclinics.com

Moving?

Make sure your subscription moves with you!

To notify us of your new address, find your **Clinics Account Number** (located on your mailing label above your name), and contact customer service at:

Email: journalscustomerservice-usa@elsevier.com

800-654-2452 (subscribers in the U.S. & Canada)
314-447-8871 (subscribers outside of the U.S. & Canada)

Fax number: 314-447-8029

Elsevier Health Sciences Division
Subscription Customer Service
3251 Riverport Lane
Maryland Heights, MO 63043

*To ensure uninterrupted delivery of your subscription, please notify us at least 4 weeks in advance of move.

Printed and bound by CPI Group (UK) Ltd, Croydon, CR0 4YY

03/10/2024

01040486-0005